ENABLING LIVES

Biographies of Six Prominent Americans with Disabilities

D1304455

ENABLING LIVES

Biographies of Six Prominent Americans with Disabilities

BRIAN T. McMAHON, Ph.D., C.R.C.
LINDA R. SHAW, Ph.D., C.R.C.

CRC Press
Boca Raton London New York Washington, D.C.

Library of Congress Cataloging-in-Publication Data

Enabling lives : biographies of six prominent americans with disabilities / edited by
Brian T. McMahon and Linda R. Shaw
  p. cm.
Includes bibliographical references.
ISBN 0-8493-0351-6 (alk. paper)
1. Handicapped—United States Biography. 2. Handicapped—Civil
rights—United States. I. McMahon, Brian T. II. Shaw, Linda R.
HV1552.3.E53   1999
362.4'092'273—dc21   99-16192
[B]

Visit the CRC Press Web site at www.crcpress.com

© 2000 by CRC Press LLC

No claim to original U.S. Government works
International Standard Book Number 0-8493-0351-6
Library of Congress Card Number 99-16192
Printed in the United States of America   2 3 4 5 6 7 8 9 0
Printed on acid-free paper

Contributors

Brian T. McMahon, Ph.D., CRC
Brian T. McMahon is a professor and chair of the rehabilitation counseling department at Virginia Commonwealth University. He has authored over 75 publications, has coedited four books on matters of employment and disability, and is a leading educator in the area of implementing the Americans with Disabilities Act. McMahon is a licensed psychologist, certified rehabilitation counselor, national certified counselor, and a certified case manager. He is a Fellow in the American Psychological Association and currently serves on the governing council of the American Counseling Association. McMahon has served on the boards of four national professional associations, including a term as president of the American Rehabilitation Counseling Association. He has received considerable recognition, including the Outstanding Rehabilitation Educator of the Year award from the National Association of Rehabilitation Professionals in the private sector; the University of Wisconsin–Milwaukee Alumni Association Award for Teaching Excellence; and the James F. Garret Career Research Award from the American Rehabilitation Counseling Association.

Al Condeluci, Ph.D.
Al Condeluci is a lifelong resident of the Pittsburgh area. He received his masters and doctorate degrees at the University of Pittsburgh. For the past 25 years, Condeluci has been associated with UCP of Pittsburgh where he currently serves as the chief executive officer. He holds faculty appointments at the University of Pittsburgh's school of health and rehabilitation sciences and the school of social work. Condeluci lectures extensively around the country, often on material from his books *Interdependence* (1991, 1995) and *Beyond Difference* (1996). He and his wife, Liz, and their children, Dante, Gianna, and Santino, live on the family "hill" in McKees Rocks, Pennsylvania with 15 other Condeluci families.

Christine Reid, Ph.D.
Christine Reid is an assistant professor in the department of rehabilitation counseling at Virginia Commonwealth University. Her experience as an educator, researcher, and service provider has focused on developing and improving structures for effective counseling and evaluation services with

people who have disabilities. Reid has published and presented rehabilitation-related topics to regional, national, and international audiences. She serves on the editorial boards of *Rehabilitation Education* and the *Journal of Counseling and Development*, as well as on the board of directors for the Commission on the Accreditation of Counseling and Related Educational Programs, representing the American Rehabilitation Counseling Association. Reid is a certified rehabilitation counselor, national certified counselor, certified vocational evaluator, certified life care planner, licensed applied psychologist (Virginia), licensed clinical professional counselor (Illinois), and licensed professional vocational rehabilitation counselor (Louisiana).

Linda R. Shaw, Ph.D., CRC

Linda R. Shaw is an associate professor at the University of Florida department of rehabilitation counseling. She has authored over 40 publications on neurologic rehabilitation, rehabilitation counseling, and disability, including two coedited books. Shaw is a certified rehabilitation counselor, a national certified counselor, and a licensed mental health counselor. She has served in multiple leadership positions with rehabilitation counseling professional associations, including having served as past president of the American Rehabilitation Counseling Association. Currently, she is a National Rehabilitation Counseling Association appointee to the Commission for Rehabilitation Counselor Certification. Shaw has also served on many volunteer boards for advocacy organizations, including several centers for independent living and state brain injury associations.

Robert T. Fraser, Ph.D., CRC

Robert T. Fraser is a professor at the University of Washington Medical Center with joint appointments in neurology, neurosurgery, and rehabilitation medicine. He is a certified rehabilitation counselor and rehabilitation psychologist. In addition to coauthoring over 60 publications and administering several successful research grants, Fraser developed a popular video series on traumatic brain injury rehabilitation. Fraser was awarded a World Rehabilitation Fund fellowship to review head injury programs in Israel. He is a two-time recipient of the prestigious Research Award of the American Rehabilitation Counseling Association. Fraser is a fellow in the American Psychology Association Division of Rehabilitation Psychology and is counted among its past presidents. He was recently elected to a four-year term at the Epilepsy Foundation of America, where he was formerly a board member.

Justin Dart, Advocate

Justin Dart, Jr. founded and was the CEO of two small businesses, one of which started with four persons and grew to 26,000 employees. He spent more than four decades of advocating for human rights in the United States, Mexico, Japan, Vietnam, Canada, Netherlands, and Germany. Dart has served five gubernatorial, one congressional, and five presidential appointments in the area of disability policy. During the past decade, he visited each of the fifty states at least five times to advocate for the passage and implementation of the historic Americans with Disabilities Act, and the empowerment of people with and without disabilities. In 1993, he resigned as chairman of the President's Committee on Employment of People with Disabilities in order to become a full-time advocate for a society that empowers all to live their God-given potential. Dart was a 1998 recipient of the nation's highest civilian award: the Presidential Medal of Freedom.

Dedication

To my mother, Jeannine Knight Shaw, who has inspired everything I have ever done that is good, or worthy, or loving.

To my father, John Robert Shaw, who proves daily the quiet power of enduring love and devotion.

Linda Shaw

To my two most wonderful children, Megan Catherine McMahon ("May-May") and Daniel Joseph McMahon ("Good Boy Dan"). You mean "only everything" to me.

Brian McMahon

Heartfelt appreciation is also extended to all six subjects for the time, cooperation, and patience required for the completion of these stories. It has been an honor and a pleasure to work with each of you: Judy, Harold, Tony, Evan, Frank, and Justin.

Linda Shaw and Brian McMahon

Contents

Foreword

It is an honor to write the foreword for *Enabling Lives*. I have personally known each of these six individuals as colleagues, friends, and mentors, and in the cases of Bowe, Dart, and Coelho, as a member of their staff. I have incredible respect and gratitude for what they have done and for the influence they have had on me.

This important book provides convincing insight into the lives and contributions of six leaders of one of the world's most profound social and human rights movements. The authors show us how Harold Russell, Evan Kemp, Justin Dart, Judy Heumann, Frank Bowe, and Tony Coelho have helped create a new paradigm in human experience: a paradigm in which we as human beings have begun to recognize that disability, whatever it is or is not, is a common occurrence within the human condition, and that it has nothing to do with being human. Through the accounts provided by the biographers, we learn less about how these six courageous individuals have overcome their disabilities to become successful, and more about how they have used their unique circumstances to create a new vision and reality for us all.

This book helps us see how these individuals have refused to let their disabilities define their lives. Instead, the reader learns how they have continued to redefine the way America and the world react to this concept called disability. We read how the efforts in their personal and professional lives have focused, with the intensity of laser beams, on maximizing the abilities inherent in us all.

These amazing biographies teach us how these six individuals have played their eminent parts in the disability rights movement, how each of them has developed a profound sense of democratic principles. and how they have all embraced the importance of extending participation in our democratic and economic processes to everyone. They are teachers of the critical realization that the strength and survival of our nation and society depends on our will, and our ability to optimize individual participation.

The biographers show how Russell, Kemp, Dart, Heumann, Bowe, and Coelho understand, and have used, the power of effective communication in the creation of a new paradigm for this concept we call disability. By the continual sharing of their vision of what is achievable for people with disabilities, they have helped create new possibilities for hundreds of millions of people worldwide. We learn how their consistent and timely communications have had momentous impact, and that they all realized that effective and calculated self-expression was their personal responsibility and their opportunity to effect change.

These are six happy and secure individuals. While they have all experienced exhilarating high points and depressing low points, personal tragedies and discrimination, and failures and successes, their happiness comes from their acceptance of life's vagaries. In all of them, it is their acceptance and their happiness that have enabled them to continually create new realities out of their visions. They possess a basic freedom from the paralysis of the past and the present in which many of us allow ourselves to get caught.

Many in our society might see these leaders as successful people struggling with serious health problems. Instead, our biographers show us six incredibly healthy individuals, as measured by their extraordinary participation and effectiveness. They are clearly not individuals who are at the mercy of their disabilities. Maybe it is because of this that this book will be the most valuable to readers with so-called disabilities. Health is ultimately measured by participation, not by diagnosis or prognosis, or someone else's perception of one's well-being.

Finally, the reader will have the tremendous realization that Russell, Kemp, Dart, Heumann, Bowe, and Coelho are loving people. This becomes clear as we learn of their consistent communication of new opportunities for each of us, and what is possible for all people. I feel honored to have worked with them and to have known their love. From this enjoyable book, I have learned things about them I had never known.

If you are looking for a feel-good, inspirational read about folks who have overcome all odds, this is not the book for you. If you are looking for insight and inspiration regarding the subject of disability, or questioning what it takes for true accomplishment, then this book is for you.

John A. Lancaster
February 15, 1999
Washington, D.C.

Introduction

The idea for this book was born one April day as my coauthor, Brian Mc-Mahon, and I were talking about the disability civil rights movement. We are both college professors and rehabilitation counselors. We were worried about whether we'd given our students a proper appreciation of the roots of the movement to secure the human rights of individuals with disabilities. That was, after all, the population they would be serving when they graduated and began working. We worried, because we knew that disability civil rights have not entered the mainstream of consciousness of most people, and our students were no exception.

One month earlier, we had celebrated Martin Luther King, Jr. Day, but where was the holiday celebrating the leaders of the disability civil rights movement? Was our movement any less notable? Less dramatic? Less worthy of recognition? Did anybody outside our own small circle of disability advocates even know the names of the heroes of our civil rights movement? On impulse, I picked up the phone and called my mother. My mom was diagnosed with multiple sclerosis nearly 40 years ago. She has lived with a progressive disability for all that time and has been heartened to see the changes in society that have made her life a little easier — curb cuts for her wheelchair, talking books, and other little changes. "Mom," I said, "who are the leaders of the disability civil rights movement?" My mother paused for several seconds and slowly said, "The what?" Now, my mother is not an uneducated or unaware person. She is a well-read woman, one of the smartest I have ever known. She couldn't come up with a name — not one.

My coauthor and I decided, on the spot, that what was needed was a book containing short biographies of some of the leaders of the disability civil rights movement. After we congratulated ourselves on our splendid idea, we started the more difficult process of figuring out who we would feature, and how we would go about getting the book done. We brainstormed and came up with a list of names. In despair, we immediately realized that it would probably take years to do the project properly. There were just too many people — and they were all too important to be left out. Finally, we decided on a strategy. We would choose six individuals and invite them to participate. We would substitute other people on the list for any who declined to participate, and if there were any names left by the time we were finished, we'd just have to plan a second volume. We started calling, and personally went to visit, each person to explain the project. Much to our surprise, every one of the chosen individuals indicated a desire to participate. We were delighted, and we definitely need to plan a second volume.

We started with Harold Russell. Harold was an absolute joy to work with, and we all became good friends, but we quickly realized that the time commitment required for each chapter would make it difficult to finish the book in a timely manner. For the first time, we considered making the book an edited work, so we selected various authors to complete each chapter. It was difficult to let go of the joy of getting to know each of our subjects, but when the chapters began to arrive, we were happy to have had the insight to involve other writers. While each chapter is written in a style that characterizes the unique approach of its author, each, in its own way, captures the life of an individual whom all Americans should look up to as a hero of the disability civil rights movement.

Though the chapters are different stylistically, they are alike in many critically important respects. Each focuses on an extraordinary American with a disability. Each of the subjects has made a significant impact on the lives of the people who have known and loved them. Each of them has engaged in activism on behalf of people with disabilities, which has changed the very social fabric of our society. And each of them deserves his or her own special place in history and in the consciousness of every American who values his or her human rights.

We present them here to you, the reader: Harold Russell, Justin Dart, Evan Kemp, Judy Heumann, Frank Bowe, and Tony Coelho, with our hopes that this book will serve as an introduction to the reader of six American heroes whose names will eventually be immediately recognized as the true heroes they are.

Linda Shaw

chapter one

Harold Russell

Brian T. McMahon

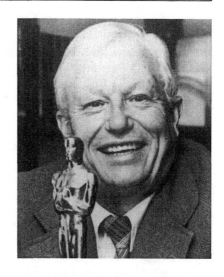

Foundation or failure?

Blanche Russell would require every bit of courage she could muster, and she had better muster it quickly. She had no choice, now that her beloved husband, only thirty-three years old, had passed away after a five-year illness. North Sydney, Nova Scotia would now have to find a new manager for its Western Union office. It was not as though Blanche had never before faced hardship — even during times of plenty, nothing had come easily to the Russell family.

By 1919, Canadian national policies had brought about a fifty-year period of booming industrialization. Particularly during those war years, the increased demand for coal meant more jobs, and the population literally exploded. The work was hard, the people rugged. The seacoast was dotted with rocky cliffs, inlets, coves, bays, and wooden houses. The area was stitched together by railroad tracks, inlet waterways, and dirt roads. Persistence. Stick-to-it-iveness. Her life in North Sydney had provided Blanche with these qualities.

After weighing her options, Blanche decided to explore the opportunities of a more diverse economy and a larger city in the United States. She joined a stream of Nova Scotians with similar inclinations, and moved to Cambridge, Massachusetts. With Bronco, their huge shaggy dog, and her three

1-57444-083-7/00/$0.00+$.50
© 2000 by CRC Press LLC

boys in tow, Harry, Les, and Bob, she settled on Antrim Street, where many neighbors and relatives had established their own Canadian colony, under the initial sponsorship of the Munn family, a group of French Canadians who had assisted many families in their relocation to the United States.

Fortunately, Blanche had a marketable skill. She had trained as a practical nurse and quickly found a job working ten or eleven hours a day for $25 per week. It was hard work, for sure, but her new life had its small pleasures. She loved the four-mile walk to St. Paul's Church, where she worshipped regularly. The kids went along, mostly for her sake. Church was boring for them, but it was important to their mother who was kind, lovable, sweet, and strong.

Harold had always wanted to take care of his mother, and now he had the chance. At only five years of age, Harold was now the man of the house. As the years passed, he grew up under the specter of Harvard University, which, although right down the street, might just as well have been on Mars. He and his neighborhood buddies spent their time perfecting the art of playing baseball, roller hockey, and kick-the-can. The guys were great friends and hung out together constantly. One neighborhood boy, Leo Deihl, had an unexplained physical deformity, but somehow they always found a role for Leo in whatever activity they were engaged in — bat boy, umpire, right fielder, or scorekeeper — something. Nobody gave his deformity much thought. Sure, Leo was always included; why wouldn't he be? Interestingly enough, Leo went on to become a primary aide to U.S. House Speaker Tip O'Neill.

Listening to the radio was a special treat in those days. But even the radio could not compare to the six-cent movies at the Central Square Theater. Harold did not go often, but when he did, it was a delight, especially on Saturday afternoons, which offered triple features and a piano player. After the show, the usher used a bamboo stick to shoo away the kids. But Harry was growing up, and his attention would eventually be diverted. Under the tutelage of Uncle Wolf (Wilfred Croucher), Harry was learning the awkward process of courting the sister of his best buddy, Charley Russell. Her name was Rita, and she was the love of his young life.

But there was always work to be done and money to be earned. Anything that could supplement his mother's modest earnings was encouraged. From the ages of five to ten, this meant winning Bible recitation contests in church (a one-dollar prize) or scavenging for milk and soda bottles (a one-cent-per-bottle redemption fee). Several years later, Harold became a club fighter. Twice each month, Harold got knocked down for a loser fee of one dollar, often at the fists of young Red Priest, whose purse as winner was three dollars. In one of these bouts, Harold was triumphant quite by accident, scoring a knockout with a near-blind, roundhouse right hook.

It was at age ten, however, that young Harold found a job that provided him with the stable income his family so desperately needed. Harold Russell scored big, landing a job delivering groceries at Lynds Grocery Store. The pay was decent — 25 cents for each delivery, plus tip (usually a nickel, but sometimes more). Each evening, he turned over ninety cents on every dollar to his appreciative mother. And so it went, year in and year out, throughout his school years at Merrill, Harvard Grammar, and Rindge Technical High School. Harold Russell had found his niche in the grocery business. When school was not in session, Harold worked every conceivable job in the grocery business. After hours, he put up stock, cleaned floors, and did whatever was needed. Weekend hours of work began at 7 A.M. and ended at 2 A.M. the following day.

Harold's future seemed secure. In 1932, as the date of his high school graduation neared, two large grocery companies merged — Ginter Company (which included Harold's store) and Arthur E. Doyle. First National Stores was the result, and rumor had it that some jobs would be lost. Harold's hopes turned to college; he wanted to attend MIT. Inspired by the Lindbergh flight and a five-minute recreational airplane ride at age seventeen, Harold dreamed of a career in aeronautical engineering, although he was not quite sure exactly what an aeronautical engineer did. Several problems stood in the way, however — poor fine-motor skills and a complete lack of funds among them. Mediocre grades in math and science ruled out the possibility of a scholarship, so his MIT dream seemed lost.

Harold's hard work and ambition in the grocery business, however, would pay dividends. Harold was not laid off, and before long, was promoted from delivery boy to a counter man in the meat department. The surly butcher, Jeff Butler, took a liking to him, and trained him in the art of meat cutting. Harold demonstrated that he could relate well to the customers, which was necessary to proceed into advanced training — which meant learning how to cut meat "at a profit." Prescribed profit margins had to be reached in order to maintain employment. Butler taught Harold the fine art of shaving weights, incorrectly adding merchandise, chicken switching, and creative weighing — all while engaged in innocent chit-chat with the customer. The right or wrong of it all never caused Harold to worry much; it was just the way things worked, since the profit margin had to be reached. Still, the thought sometimes crossed his mind — would there someday be retribution for such cheap practices?

Having shown a sincere appreciation for the profit margin, Harold was given the opportunity to become a relief manager, and eventually a special manager who opened up new stores for the chain and oriented incoming managers. He enjoyed his increases in responsibility and authority, and by age twenty-five was earning $40 per week, plus "a few steaks" — more than he had ever dared imagine. Additional dollars were earned by recruiting members for the American Meatcutters of North America. Another dollar or two was earned in the quiet distribution of illegal whiskey. The money was faithfully forwarded to Blanche for management of the family's needs.

Labor relations in the meat cutters' unions were very intense during those years. Two particularly active unions were the Amalgamated Butcher Workers and the American Meatcutters of North America. Both were eager to gain a foothold in the growing business of chain stores in Massachusetts, and a high priority was organizing the employees of the meat departments at the First National Stores. Harold Russell invited fellow workers to attend organizing meetings and drove prospects to and from the gatherings.

One Wednesday morning, two senior managers, William Lynds and Joseph McCarthy, invited Harold into the office, which was actually the walk-in refrigerator of the grocery chain — a very private, cold, and frightening place. Harold was anxious, cold, and shaking, as McCarthy pressed, "Where were you last night?" "At the movies," lied Harold, seeing his job, life, and family's future on the line. "You were at a union meeting," accused McCarthy. He was given an ultimatum: he could resign from either the company or from the union within two weeks. Six days later, as Harold agonized over the matter, a federal law was passed prohibiting management from taking adverse personnel actions against employees involved with recognized, legal unions. Once again, Harold Russell was saved.

As a young man, Harold had a longstanding dream of acquiring "wheels." In a deliberate, wishful manner, he squirreled away a dollar here and there while undertaking a thorough investigation of the automobile market. Eventually, he found a used Model A Ford for $250 — $50 down and $50 per month. He had no idea how he would make the payments, but the deal was consummated. The dream of a lifetime was realized, and suddenly Harold was "Mister Big" among his comrades.

He had no shortage of friends now. Showing off his new car included driving to Boston with four buddies, with Harold at the wheel. At the end of Broadway, just before the bridge over the Charles River, was Boston's infamous rotary. To the horror of his passengers, the car skidded and overturned due to Harold's inattention. No one was even scratched, but the fear of those awful moments lasted a lifetime. From this experience, Harold Russell developed a sense of invulnerability that would influence his subsequent decisions to volunteer for duty where others feared to tread.

Harold Russell's early work years molded his future. His arsenal of personal resources now included specialized vocational skills such as meat cutting; interpersonal and persuasive skills learned as counter man and union organizer; organizational and leadership skills developed in various management positions; and program development skills honed as development manager. Personal responsibility and hard work were Harold's prized values. At every turn, there was also the aggressive pursuit of more compensation, responsibility, and authority. These experiences would serve him well in his subsequent military, filmmaking, and political careers.

An astute observer of Harold's development might have noticed his increasing propensity for risk taking. He constantly jeopardized secure positions by seizing daring opportunities to maximize income, such as incorrectly weighing meat, "borrowing" steaks, bootlegging, and organizing workers from his management position. From time to time, he would risk it all — for money, excitement, or principle. Harold Russell was a restless young man.

Soldiering and the great adventure

As a young adult, Harold Russell was becoming burned out. After eighteen years in the grocery business, his opportunities for advancement were drying up. His union organizing and occasional bootlegging activities left him searching for more excitement. He was frustrated that he had not realized his dream of becoming an aeronautical engineer. It seemed to Harold that he had failed at school, at sports, and in his long-term career pursuits. Could it be that at only twenty-five years of age he had peaked? Was this all there was?

Harold had also failed at love. Rita married Richard Nixon, a long-time schoolmate and competitor of his. The news from Charley of her marriage had literally sickened Harold. In February 1942, all of his hopes and dreams were shattered by the wedding. He heard rumblings that Rita's marriage was less than ideal, but this gossip offered little comfort. Harold Russell sought escape.

Pearl Harbor provided an obvious solution — the universal call to arms. Harold's draft status had been deferred, as the primary supporter of his mother. The new national commitment appealed to Harold Russell who was seeking to perform his patriotic duty, by pursuing immediate enlistment. He approached the Navy, Army, Marines, and Canadian Air Corps, but was rejected as medically unfit in each attempt, due to an impacted wisdom tooth. Like other young men in this position, Harold was very embarrassed.

After a while, the acceleration of America's involvement in the war led to greater flexibility in the military's definition of what constituted adequate health for a recruit. In February 1942, Harold's mother reported to him that his brother Bob would be able to care for her while Harold was away. Harold Russell was ordered to report for basic infantry training at Camp Croft, near Spartanburg, South Carolina. After eight weeks, PFC Russell was earning $21 per month, a far cry from the $35 per week he had earned prior to enlistment, but Harold was quite content with the discipline of the Army life. It provided him with an escape from his banal existence at the grocery store and from a lifetime of perceived failures and mediocrity. Here, he could get a clean start and demonstrate his courage. Here, he could find adventure, excitement, thrills, honor, action — even glory! Perhaps he could even make Rita regret she had married Nixon. The thought made him smile, and he was encouraged by her regular letters suggesting that her marriage was a disappointment.

Referred to as a "Yankee bastard" by his predominantly Southern comrades, PFC Russell made sure he paid his cigarette debt immediately upon receipt of his salary. The balance of his funds was gone after less than 30 minutes at the craps table. Intrigued by games of chance, PFC Russell was amazed by the same dozen soldiers who were consistent winners, day in and day out. When basic pay was raised to $50 per month, at least some financial relief was in sight.

On Harold's last day of basic training, an unknown officer explained to the troops a new initiative to develop an American paratroop service to match, and eventually surpass, the capabilities of the German military. PFC Russell's dream of working with airplanes was resurrected. He might not be able to fly planes, but at least he could jump from them! Harold's excitement increased with the possibility, and he listened distractedly while the officer enumerated the many dangers of paratrooper training and service. With equal vigor, the recruiter discussed the requirements — brains, courage, ruggedness, guts, stamina, and courage. He said the paratrooper would be God's perfect man — tougher, rougher, uglier, harder, faster, smarter, stronger, and bolder than any other soldier in this, or any other, army! Harold felt a moment of confusion; first, he thought of Rita's expression when she saw those silver wings signifying membership in this "elite" branch of the United States Army, then he had a moment of hesitation and anxiety. The recruiter continued his pitch, explaining that volunteers would receive an *additional $50 per month of hazardous duty pay*! At the conclusion of the officer's remarks, PFC Russell was the first to volunteer. The paratroop lieutenant congratulated him with these words: "Soldier, you'll never live tó regret this." For days, Harold wondered precisely what that meant.

The training took place at Fort Benning, Georgia, where in the next thirty days, the newly promoted Corporal Russell completed four static line jumps and one free jump. The training was rugged and attrition exceeded 50%. A man washed out at the slightest infraction, hesitation, or sign of weakness. In spite of the challenges, the civilian world had taught Corporal Russell the value of specialized job skills. With this in mind, and attracted by the lure of still another $25-per-month raise for hazardous duty, Corporal Russell completed a subsequent two-week training program in the handling of military explosives. At last, he could afford the tailor-made uniform and silk gabardine shirt that he flaunted on his coveted leaves to Atlanta. He was, after all, a 28-year-old single man in excellent health, whose normal life span might well be limited by the hazards of duty. He reasoned that he might as well live as hard as he could now. Along the way, Harold learned how to destroy power plants, bridges, trains, trucks, cars, tanks, jeeps, boats, motorcycles, half-tracks, transportation centers, and anything else of potential strategic value to the enemy. As Harold puts it:

> On July 11, 1942, I graduated from Demo school, and I
> was handed a handsome diploma which testified to my
> knowledge and skill in the science and/or art of destroy-
> ing my fellow human beings and their property.

Corporal Russell was now a part of an elite unit. When the European invasion began, he fully expected to parachute in behind enemy lines "to cause confusion, disaster, and death to the enemy" until ground troops arrived. A cadre of high-ranking French officers arrived to tour Camp Benning and evaluate the readiness of its much-ballyhooed paratroop unit. In a lightning-quick demonstration, Harold's group made a dangerously low, 300-foot jump, and blew up a bridge. This was followed by an unusual parade in which Harold and others were recycled behind the stage to exaggerate the number of trained demolitionists and re-paraded four times before the French visitors. While successful in their deception of the visiting officers, the need for rapid training of additional, qualified troops was obvious.

With the explosives training and parading complete, Corporal Russell was eager to see action. However, the need for training thousands of additional recruits in the skills of jumping and demolition took priority. Harold Russell received special orders assigning him to a stateside location as a demolition instructor. Disappointed with the assignment, but now a staff sergeant, Russell began his career as a teacher. In a short time, much to his surprise, he found this activity to be varied, interesting, and exciting. His repeated requests for transfer to an outfit located in an overseas theater of operations were denied. For the next two years, Russell taught his lessons, again and again, to classes of 100, which included 25 officers per class. In a prelude to what became his powerful public-speaking skills, Russell developed a number of attention-getting instructional techniques, including "accidentally" dropping what the trainees believed to be live TNT. To keep his jumping skills sharp, Russell completed 51 free jumps. He became a senior instructor and was now earning a respectable $153 per month.

In the first seven months of his teaching tenure, 11 of 18 instructors were injured. Harold Russell was among the first, sustaining eye damage. Then, in a foiled demonstration jump, Harold's parachute became entangled with an equipment chute, which barely supported both the human and non-human cargoes to a safe landing. Omen after omen appeared, and the fear of re-injury was everywhere, exceeded only by the fear of being injured stateside, rather than in overseas combat. Still, his repeated requests for transfer to a combat outfit were denied.

Eventually, Russell's commanding officer, Captain Phillips, was assigned to a combat outfit. Only then was Russell's request for combat duty approved. On January 12, 1944, Russell reported to the 515th Parachute Infantry Regiment of the 13th Airborne Division at Camp Mackall, near Fayetteville, North Carolina. In spite of a series of mishaps, the rugged training intensified. The commanding general was killed in a plane crash, eight troopers drowned in a lake during a training jump, and a plane collided with an equipment chute, crashing with eighteen soldiers aboard.

The plane crash directly involved Staff Sergeant Russell. It was a Friday night, and Russell was bringing his class back from the field in a small truck. Night jumps on Fridays were routine, and he hurried to connect with a particular plane where his close friend and roommate was the jumpmaster. The two friends had planned to drink a few beers after the exercise. On the way, the truck suddenly lurched and the driver reported a flat tire, which was hurriedly changed. As the truck finally approached the airstrip, Staff Sergeant Russell could see his intended flight take off. Dismayed, he instructed the driver to return the class to the school area, and he sat down to watch the jump. That way the two buddies could at least compare notes after the brief exercise.

The C-47 made the routine turn into the jump zone and veered to the right. Suddenly, it headed straight for the ground, and in a matter of seconds — which seemed like forever— it crashed and burst into flames. Staff Sergeant Russell rushed to the crash site, but was driven back by the intense heat of the plane, which was still exploding and burning wildly. He could hear the screams of the soldiers inside. Waiting for the wreckage to cool, it struck him that his life had been spared by a flat tire. Reminded of the Model A Ford accident, Russell marveled at how God works in strange and mysterious ways. His inner sense of invulnerability and good fortune was further reinforced.

The big bang

It was June 1944. New and demanding infiltration courses were set up involving rugged terrain, live explosives and ammunition, and sniper fire. This was all okay with Staff Sergeant Harold Russell, because soon he would finally see action.

The heat and humidity in North Carolina were relentless and Staff Sergeant Russell was restless beyond words. Deployment abroad was imminent. In recent days, three train trips to the coast for overseas transfer had been canceled at the last minute. However, full mobilization was now expected in a matter of hours. Rumors abounded regarding the scope and risks of the pending mission. Believing the rumors were true, Harold wrote and mailed what he felt might be his last letter — a "Dear John" letter to his girlfriend Rita, recently divorced from Nixon at last — a letter releasing her to find another partner.

Stateside, Russell had one final job to do. He had been asked to supervise the preparation of a new, more rigorous infiltration course — one that would give the outfit more experience with explosives. Until deployment, 1000 troops per day would run the 1500-yard course littered with cut-out targets and four-ounce plastic explosives. Although the plastique was presumed to be as safe, or safer, than the more familiar TNT, the training occurred in a field fifteen miles outside Camp Mackall. The pressure of the assignment was enormous and was intensified by the hot climate and the anticipation. Having worked hard on the layout, Staff Sergeant Russell was scheduled to have the next week off for a much-deserved rest. That was the week Sergeant Stutzman had been assigned to run the demolition platoon, but Stutzman needed a favor, because his girl was coming to visit for a few days. Although wracked by fatigue and the anticipation of shipping out, Russell agreed to pinch hit for his old pal.

Staff Sergeant Russell had been raised in the Episcopalian faith, but he was not a deeply religious man. However, this was one period in his life when he appreciated the comfort of his spiritual beliefs. The training experiences, which included free-fall parachute jumps and live ammunition, suddenly brought God into focus for him. On this day, which would soon be known as D-Day, Staff Sergeant Russell keenly felt his more typical exasperation with religion.

It was the morning of June 6, 1944. Right after reveille, it was announced that paratroopers had spearheaded an allied invasion of Europe. Everyone was excited, and Russell's unit went to work setting and planting the 500 charges required for the morning training session. Russell began his normal routine — supervising this activity, and indicating where each charge was to be set. All was well, and the entire First Battalion completed the course by noon. At noon, the frenetic pace of preparations was interrupted by the chaplain, who provided an update on the Normandy invasion. Unaware of the battalion's current assignment, the chaplain embellished the announcement, talking for more than an hour, adding personal sentiments, invocations, and prayers.

Although the announcement elevated his excitement to a new level, Staff Sergeant Russell's mind was not on the action overseas. He could only think of preparing the infiltration course, which was scheduled to resume at 1300 hours, and was falling farther and farther behind. The European campaign had begun, and they would be leaving any day now, at any hour. The outfit had been alerted, and time was short. Preparing these fine men was his job, and as with every previous expectation of him, he intended to do it right, and on time. The chaplain's sermon was unnecessary and unscheduled. It was not supposed to happen that way.

As the chaplain droned on, the caps for the explosives lay exposed in the sun, increasing their sensitivity, and therefore, increasing the risks associated with their handling. A military inquiry later revealed that for one particular cap, the additional sun exposure compounded a defect that had gone undetected by production inspectors. It was not supposed to happen that way.

When the chaplain departed, the preparations resumed. Staff Sergeant Russell was frustrated and angered by the delay. Back at the training course, a brushfire had been started by one of the charges. It was promptly extinguished, but Russell was now an hour behind schedule.

As they hurried, one soldier was having an inordinate degree of difficulty in setting his charge. Under normal circumstances, Staff Sergeant Russell would have walked him through it, troubleshooting the problem — collectively solving it, correcting it, and reviewing the lessons learned. There was no time for that now — it was already 1:30 P.M. Russell decided to just pitch in himself and help the boys prepare the charges. It was not supposed to happen that way.

With a desperate urgency, Russell was reflexively prepping charges at a frantic pace — nearly one per minute. Break off half a pound of nitrostarch, insert a fuse into a cap, crimp them together, jam them into the explosive, tape them in securely...

Evacuation

Russell never lost consciousness. Immediately following the explosion, the first words he heard, loud and clear, were, "There goes the great Russell." He observed the whole situation in all of its ugliness, and every moment passed in slow motion until he was anesthetized for surgery. There was blood everywhere. Tourniquets, sulfa, and blankets were applied. Drugs were given. Staff Sergeant Russell was moved gently, but quickly, into the chaplain's jeep for the fifteen-mile scurry to the base hospital. Curiously, there was no pain, just a mild stinging of his arms and stomach. He looked at his arms. His hands were gone, and in their place were bloody shreds of skin, muscle, and bone. His chest and stomach were bleeding. Staff Sergeant Russell never lost consciousness. It was not supposed to happen that way.

Two life-saving forces intervened. The first was Harold's combat attire, which included a special vest for explosives. The second involved two men. The jeep was slowed to a crawl by an elaborate traffic entanglement. Men, equipment, and vehicles littered the road from the demolition training site to the base hospital, a distance of about ten miles. Medical emergencies in transit were not anticipated, and certainly not by jeep. The jeep driver and the escorts had all but given up hope.

Out of nowhere, two motorcycles ridden by MPs appeared and almost struck Staff Sergeant Russell's vehicle. In an instant, the MPs evaluated the situation and took action. One man cleared the traffic to accelerate the trip to the base hospital, and the other drove ahead to alert the surgical team. Within twenty minutes, Staff Sergeant Russell was being prepared for surgery by appropriate medical personnel with the proper emergency equipment. This fast response time was more consistent with the techniques of modern-day paramedics and life flight. Staff Sergeant Russell would never learn the names of those instinctive MPs, who just happened by and expedited transport. It was not supposed to happen that way.

Staff Sergeant Russell's surgery required two hours. Both hands were amputated approximately two inches above the wrist. Black powder was washed from his eye sockets, but some would remain forever. The noise of the explosion caused permanent, partial deafness to his left ear. But the surgeons' greatest concern was the damage to his abdomen, which was entirely blown open. Even after the obvious repairs, the risk of infection from residual powder remained high. Sergeant Russell survived his injuries. It was not supposed to happen that way.

When Staff Sergeant Russell awoke, his arms were in traction above him on pulleys. To his intense horror, he observed that he had no hands at the ends of his arms. "As long as I live," he said to himself, "there will be no hands!" Immediately, he thought the unthinkable: he did not want to live. There could be no life without hands! The medical staff conveyed that their greater concerns were with his life-threatening abdominal injuries. Suddenly, his hands seemed more dispensable, and life seemed worth living again. In the future, there would be little consideration given to suicide.

The Great Adventure, World War II, continued, but without Staff Sergeant Harold Russell. Ironically, it was this very same "act of God" that actually allowed him to survive the war. Harold Russell's misfortune had been great, but not as great as that of his own unit. The 515th Airborne was dispatched to Europe to further the momentum of the D-Day invasion. In September 1944, Operation Market Garden began. It was an ill-fated campaign, designed by General Montgomery to bring an early end to World War II by Christmas. The plan required 35,000 men to be flown 300 miles and dropped behind enemy lines. Harold Russell's unit of 1500 paratroopers, with demolition capabilities, was a part of that campaign; it was the largest airborne operation ever mounted. In one of the greatest intelligence boondoggles in military history, several thousand paratroopers had been dropped, in daylight, directly upon two SS Panzer divisions commanded by General Bittrich. Casualties on that day alone exceeded 90%.

Today, Harold Russell views himself as a very fortunate man. Foremost among his regrets, however, is that he never experienced combat. It was a matter of ability utilization. His highly specialized combat skills, developed over a period of three years, were never put to use in the field of valor. Even worse, in his mind, was that his wartime injuries had not been received in combat. Given the extraordinary public exposure he eventually received, most admirers presumed that his injuries were combat related. While he never contributed to this inaccuracy, Harold always felt a measure of guilt about it, which may have led, albeit subconsciously, to his early refusal of additional motion-picture opportunities, and his general avoidance of the limelight. In his own words, "I was blown up on the wrong side of the ocean."

Russell's private D-Day

Staff Sergeant Harold Russell was stabilized at the Camp Mackall base hospital, and stayed for nine days. From there, he was transferred to Walter Reed Hospital for additional surgery, prosthetics, and rehabilitation services. Staff Sergeant Russell was placed in Ward 32, an amputee ward with 42 patients. Over the next several months, Harold gradually realized that life would go on. He cites several experiences that were important to his eventual recovery. First and foremost among these was the friendliness and camaraderie of his fellow patients. All were similarly situated; they were young soldiers who had received significant disabilities in the course of their military duties. Their shared experience created an immediate bond, whose therapeutic effects were unmatched in civilian life. The opportunity to observe and interact with other successful rehabilitants, particularly veterans like himself who were "making it," helped define the possibilities and provided a flicker of hope for the future. Tony Falbo, a fellow patient with bilateral amputation of the upper extremities, was particularly close to Harold.

Ward 32 was an environment characterized by humor and storytelling. Practical jokes, involving direct exploitation of the target's impairment, were rampant. Learning to laugh at himself paid dividends that would benefit

Harold for a lifetime. The hospital provided aggressive, state-of-the-art physical rehabilitation techniques. Prosthetics, orthotics, physical therapy, and
occupational therapy services were first-rate, and reality factors and functional activities were emphasized.

But the psychological adjustment was difficult, especially at night:

> ...When I was alone and the big ward was quiet and
> dark, the long, heavy thoughts would come marching
> back into my mind. Then I would start thinking about
> the future, wondering what I was going to do, how I
> was going to get along when they discharged me from
> the Army, and I'd be on my own again on the Outside.
> The Outside was already beginning to worry and
> frighten me...going out there alone, without hands.
> Would they give me a break? Would they be morbidly
> inquisitive? Would they be indifferent? I had no idea
> and I was afraid of that grim day when I would have
> to leave the cloistered shelter of the hospital to find
> out for myself.

Harold had too much time to ruminate. Ruminate about discharge. Ruminate
about the cosmetic hand vs. functional, but ghastly, hooks. Ruminate about
making a living. Ruminate about being unable to perform both necessary
and fun activities, as before. Ruminate about becoming dependent on someone else for assistance with personal care and hygiene. Ruminate about how
his friends, family, and Rita would react to him. Worse yet, was the rumination about why — why this had happened to him:

> I used to lie awake for hours, thinking and wondering
> and wishing and going over all those tremendous *ifs*
> in my mind. *If* I hadn't taken over Stutzman's assign-
> ment — *If* Eisenhower hadn't postponed D-Day from
> June 5 to June 6 because of bad weather over the En-
> glish Channel — *If* the chaplain hadn't come out to
> brief us — *If* there hadn't been a brushfire — *If* I hadn't
> pitched in to help the boys with preparing the charges
> — *If* — *If* — *If*.

The rumination and the nights were torturing Russell. It was a long and
difficult battle:

> ...When the shadows lengthened and darkness came,
> I began to waver and wonder, and to question myself.
> Perhaps one reason for that was the fact that I had not
> yet become reconciled to my state of handlessness. I
> stubbornly refused to accept it or to make the necessary

mental adjustments. I still kept hoping against hope
that in some vague, miraculous way I would sprout a
new pair of hands overnight.

More difficult times lay ahead. As the doctors began deliberations about his
discharge, he had visitors, community outings, and home visits. These activities created fear and panic in Staff Sergeant Russell, reminiscent of his first
parachute jump. Harold lingered at the hospital, seeking to avoid "the
inquisitive questions of well-meaning strangers, the naked stares of barflies,
and the self-conscious embarrassment of everyone I met." Harold still struggled with the psychological problems, comparing and contrasting the new
and the old Harold, and viewing every human interaction with suspicion
bordering on paranoia. Representative of these experiences was the following vignette about a flight attendant who had just reminded Harold to
unfasten his safety belt:

> I started to pull my hooks out of my pockets, but they
> got stuck. I wrestled with them for a few seconds, and
> finally I got them out after nearly ripping off my pants.
> Then I began fumbling with the belt. She had offered
> to close it before we took off, but I had declined stiffly.
> Now she stood over me like a schoolteacher, watching
> me struggle with it. I just couldn't seem to get a grip
> on that slippery metal buckle. I could almost hear her
> saying, "See! What did I tell you? You can't do it by
> yourself." That only made me more nervous. Finally
> she reached down, flipped it open and walked off tri-
> umphantly into the cockpit. I fell back against the seat.
> This was the ultimate humiliation. Only a few months
> before I had been the rough, tough paratrooper, boldly
> leaping into the wild blue yonder...

Harold's old fears about retribution for the sins of his youth resurfaced.
Eventually, though, he was able to view this concern with sardonic humor:

> One morning I met a woman who had been one of my
> good customers in the meat market..."You know,
> Harold, I wouldn't worry too much over those hands,"
> she said, "they never really belonged to you...every
> time you weighed meat you sold part of them."

Harold was convinced that Rita would be better off without him. He felt she
should take up with somebody "whole." Their relationship became rocky
as Harold attempted to terminate it by using persuasion, deliberate ignoring,
and subterfuge. Rita would have none of it. She stood by him through all
his obnoxious tantrums and antics. She was steadfast, further contributing

to Harold's fears. He longed to stay at Walter Reed, where no one bothered him, hounded him, nagged him, or heckled him about his plans for the future. He enjoyed the peace and understanding he received there, even if it was not the "real world."

Occupational therapy helped. Four hours a day, under the close super-vision of Miss Schram, Harold Russell studied numerous subjects, until he passed a proficiency exam. They included dressing, eating, writing, shaving, tying his shoelaces, dialing a phone, brushing his teeth, typing, playing ping pong, handling faucets, smoking, drinking, shooting pool, blowing his nose, turning book pages, playing checkers, handling coins. Nothing came easy! Mastering these lessons, however, helped with his mental adjustments. Learning how to conserve energy by properly planning and sequencing his activities helped even more.

Harold was tireless in the execution of his rehabilitation program. He appreciated the devotion and commitment of his therapists. Still, he occa-sionally resented receiving instructions from people with hands, no matter how qualified. He gradually modified the lessons to suit his own individual circumstances. After two months, Harold viewed an old training film entitled *Meet McGonegal*. The movie depicted Charley McGonegal, who had lost both hands in World War I, successfully negotiating a typical day with the adept use of his hooks. McGonegal had gotten married, made a fortune in real estate, and retired to the profitable business of breeding horses.

> The film was only five minutes long, but it "...gave me a real lift...It was the most exciting movie I had ever seen...if he could do it, I could do it, too." Thus it happened, for when it came to Sgt. Russell's real prob-lem of mental adjustment, no amount of therapy was as helpful as witnessing the successful rehabilitation of a similarly situated veteran.

Three days later, quite by surprise, Charley McGonegal visited Ward 32 at Walter Reed Hospital. Visiting daily for two weeks, he and Harold Russell became immediate friends. In an illustration of what rehabilitation philoso-phers call "residual assets," Charley emphasized to Harold that "It's not what you have lost that is important. Rather, it's what you have left that counts, and how you use it." McGonegal told Russell that self-perception and support counted most, and Harold could have both as soon as he left the "pity party" behind. He explained that Harold was lucky, that he could learn to use his amputation to his advantage.

Charley taught Harold the specifics of negotiating life without hands. Harold confessed to Charley his discomfort in social situations. Charley told him that when he met someone, he should "take those hooks and shake them in their face — make them shake your hooks. Would you ever forget shaking hands with a person who had hooks instead of hands?" While allowing Harold to make up his own mind, Charley demonstrated the many advantages of hooks vs. cosmetic hands. The two discussed issues that modern-day rehabilitation professionals consider critical to success, e.g., reality factors, individual approaches, and an acceptance of necessary assistance. Harold Russell later recalled that his encounter with Charley was the real turning point in his rehabilitation. Once again, God had saved Harold Russell — this time sending an angel named Charley.

Harold and Charley discussed famous people who had managed severe disabilities: Edison, Lord Nelson, Franklin Roosevelt, Steinmetz, Helen Keller, Beethoven, Sarah Bernhardt, and Milton. Roosevelt, in particular, was an inspiration. People either admired and loved him, or hated him, but no one ever pitied him. McGonegal and Russell began to run the numbers. They discussed how being among a couple of hundred bilateral-hand amputees, in a population of 140 million Americans, made them unique. Harold began to conquer his own doubts and fears. He began to feel ready for discharge. Charley was his role model, and his words made sense; they were the challenge that Harold had needed. They gave him a path for living. He describes Charley McGonegal as "an angel," and his visit as "food for a starving man." There was no going back now; neither rehabilitation nor life would ever be the same, thanks to Charley McGonegal. McGonegal later ran for governor of California. He lost by 800 votes.

To help conquer his fears and self-consciousness, Harold forced himself to be polite when people inquired about his hooks. By doing so, he discovered some interesting patterns. Yesterday, these people had seemed morbid and inquisitive; now they seemed genuinely interested in him. Yesterday, they had wanted to buy him a drink as an act of cheap charity; today, they were acknowledging a debt that they owed to all who had served their country. One stranger who inquired about the hooks was simply seeking guidance for his own injured son, who was wrestling with the decision about hooks vs. cosmetic hands. Harold discovered that when he talked about his hooks calmly, with detachment, and without embarrassment, nervousness, or anger, he was the center of attention. According to Harold, "That did delicious things for my sadly deflated ego."

Coming home via Hollywood

Harold began to consider a variety of careers that had little to do with the use of one's hands. Law, politics, social service, or writing were possibilities. Sales seemed even more attractive. He made plans to use the G.I. Bill to attend Boston University, and to take an advertising course at the School of Business Administration. In the meantime, Harold became so proficient in the use of his metal hooks that he was cast in an update of the McGonegal film, entitled *Diary of a Sergeant*. Harold viewed this as a useful project that would provide a temporary diversion. The movie was produced by Captain Julian Blaustein, directed by Captain Joe Newman, and filmed by Sergeant Meredith Nicholson. Instead of being a dry film demonstrating how Russell operated his hooks, the four decided to make a mini-drama, with Russell starring as the hero. It was an almost-day-by-day account of everything that had happened to him, from the time of his accident, to his going home, entering school, and starting a new life.

Russell enjoyed making *Diary of a Sergeant*. The crew filmed at Walter Reed Hospital, at Paramount Studios in New York, and on campus at Boston University. From November 1944, until the final scene was shot on New Year's Day 1945, Russell accomplished something constructive — not in spite of his impairment, but because of it. *Diary of a Sergeant* was released in March. The movie was three times longer (at twenty-four minutes) and three times more expensive (at $75,000) than originally planned. It was so successful, however, that it was used around the country at rallies to sell war bonds, and Russell was called upon to make hundreds of appearances on behalf of the bond campaign. On January 3, 1945, Harold Russell was honorably discharged from the Army. He returned to Boston, began his full-time studies, and worked at the Cambridge YMCA, running athletic programs for boys.

The Best Years of Our Lives was the first major motion picture to feature a disabled person in a key role. When *Diary of a Sergeant* was seen by Samuel Goldwyn and director William Wyler, himself a veteran, it was determined that Russell photographed well and looked younger than his years. Wyler decided then and there to screen test Harold Russell for *The Best Years of Our Lives*. Wyler and Goldwyn were advised that the country would not want to be reminded of the tragic disabilities caused by World War II so soon after its conclusion. Disregarding this advice, Wyler rewrote the script for Harold Russell, transforming the disabling condition to amputation from spasticity, as it had appeared in MacKinlay Kantor's book, *Glory for Me*, upon which the movie was based.

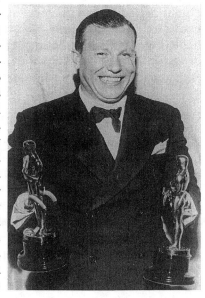

Harold Russell was the only amateur in a cast that included Frederic March, Teresa Wright, Myrna Loy, and Dana Andrews. His character was Homer Parrish, a handless sailor plagued by the double-barreled problem of readjusting to civilian life and reconnecting with his childhood sweetheart, a part that Harold could easily identify with. Amateur or not, Harold Russell received two Academy Awards for a single role, an unmatched achievement to this day. The first was a special Oscar for "bringing aid and comfort to disabled veterans through the medium of motion pictures"; the second was for Best Actor in a Supporting Role. His competition were Charles Coburn, Claude Rains, Clifton Webb, and William Demarest. Jack Benny presented the awards, and Harold accepted his second Oscar on behalf of all the veterans who had served their country in World War II. Cary Grant was among the first to congratulate Harold, adding, "Do you know where I can get some dynamite?" A young Kirk Douglas asked if Russell favored method acting. Harold replied, "What's that?"

The Best Years of Our Lives swept the 1947 Academy Awards, winning nine Oscars, including Best Picture, and the Irving G. Thalberg Award. Other best-picture nominees included *It's a Wonderful Life, Henry V, The Razor's Edge,* and *The Yearling. The Best Years of Our Lives* became the highest-grossing movie of its time, and continues to play all over the world on a regular basis.

Harold Russell quickly became an international symbol of courage in the face of adversity. For decades to come, disabled veterans of every war approached Russell, stating that the picture precisely captured the emotions and issues of re-entry which they had experienced. "That was my story," they would proclaim. Indeed, the re-entry and rehabilitation aspects of the picture remain relevant to this day.

Harold Russell fell in love with movie-making. But his love life had improved on several counts. On February 27, 1946, in the midst of shooting *The Best Years of Our Lives,* Russell married Rita. Contrary to everything he had been told, he found "film folks" to be inherently decent, generous, and friendly. While in Los Angeles to attend the Academy Awards ceremony, two scripts were presented to Harold Russell for his consideration. He admired famed director William Wyler for his hard-nosed, direct, military manner on the set. Seeking Wyler's counsel at a private dinner, Russell discussed the ups and downs of a full-time acting career. The two speculated about the potential number and quality of future roles for an actor with his impairments. Discouraged by Wyler, Russell chose not to pursue acting on a full-time basis, and returned to Boston University to pursue full-time studies in psychology on the G.I. Bill. An average student, Russell's strongest academic performances were in the area of public speaking. He graduated in 1949, and published his autobiography, *Victory in My Hands,* the same year. It was eventually translated into twenty languages.

Not since Uncle Wolf and Charley McGonegal had Russell found a mentor so helpful as William Wyler, director of such classics as *Wuthering Heights, The Memphis Belle, The Heiress, Mrs. Miniver, Dodsworth,* and *The Letter.* On December 31, 1946, Russell received a telegram from Wyler that illustrates their relationship, as well as Harold's achievements in *Best Years:*

> Dear Russ: I didn't write you before because I could never find the right words to tell you what I feel for you, but I wish you could have been here last night to see the Beverly Hills opening of *The Best Years of Our Lives* and to hear for yourself some of the glowing things that were said about the picture and about you. The New York opening was a great thrill and the re-

views were all that we could have expected and more, but last night the people who saw the picture were among the most gifted and knowing movie-makers and their sincere tributes made it as great a day for me as the day when I first saw you in *Diary of a Sergeant*. It should be a source of great satisfaction to you that by your example you are going to help so many men find a way out of their own problems. In addition, I am convinced the inspiration of your performance will reach millions of people in all countries and do untold good. No amount of hard work would have enabled you to reflect the full and splendid value of the character of Homer, if you had not been the wonderful guy you are. I can only express my deepest gratitude for what your job, so well done, has meant to the picture and to me personally. You have every right to the inner rewards and inner satisfaction which will most certainly come to you. I wish you the fullest joy in these rewards and in your own pride and knowledge that you have accomplished something so meaningful and important. With warmest regards to you and your wife, always — William Wyler.

For the next several months, Russell did promotional tours for *The Best Years of Our Lives*. There were scores of public appearances, and interviews for radio, newspapers, and magazines. Russell used these opportunities to talk about what it meant for him to be an American citizen in a free and democratic society. He broadened and deepened his own thinking as he spoke. He spoke boldly about the intolerance he had observed in his travels, and of the inconsistency of "second-class citizenship" in a democratic America. He spoke out against discrimination and prejudice between races, religions, and social classes. He articulated the status of veterans, and people with disabilities, and their difficulties in community re-entry. He appealed for better education, and better legislation to guarantee to all Americans the basic rights and privileges of citizenship. He asked people to think for themselves, and reject "party lines" and "isms" — to analyze, to weigh, to ponder, and to study everything you hear, read, and see. He advised people to take nothing for granted, and to accept no one's word on anything.

When promoting the movie ran its course, his talent and message were discovered by the Anti-Defamation League, which sponsored Harold in delivering seven weekly talks to school groups. This was a labor of love. To this day, he enjoys speaking to school groups. After a recent presentation, a spry young boy asked him, "Is there anything you can't do?" Harold paused, thought for a moment, and replied, "Why no, I don't think so." The youngster pressed on: "Do you know how to break dance?"

His most memorable speech, however, was at Soldier's Field in Chicago on October 20, 1947, at a ceremony in honor of the first war dead being returned from the Pacific. An excerpt follows:

> I wonder what they would say here if they could stand before you and speak to you, as I do now. I feel certain they would tell you to forget all the high, resounding phrases that have been uttered so many, many times before — phrases that mean little or nothing now — phrases that have never meant very much, really. I think they would say to you, men and women of America: 'Keep faith with us! Make sure that we have not died for nothing. Make sure the work we began is finished. Pray — work — fight — to build a nation that will stand, united and strong and beautiful, that will work for peace always, that will give the world that faith, that hope and leadership it so desperately needs. This is your duty to us, the war dead of America.

Russell dabbled in show business for the next forty years. Under contract to the William Morris theatrical agency in New York, he played nightclubs as a storyteller and piano player. He was the opening act for Jackie Gleason in Chicago and Vic Damone in Buffalo. In 1980, he co-starred in the Richard Donner film, *Inside Moves*, and later did guest spots in TV episodes of *Trapper John* and *China Beach*. Contrary to popular opinion, Harold felt then and continues today to characterize all of his acting associates as "nice people."

In and around the White House

In 1947, in the midst of his college studies, Harold Russell received a request from President Harry Truman to join the newly formed President's Committee on the Employment of the Physically Handicapped. As a veteran soldier, he was not about to refuse the commander in chief. In this capacity, Russell chaired a committee for veterans' issues. In 1962, he was appointed vice chairman by President John F. Kennedy; two years later he was appointed chairman by President Lyndon Johnson. He served in this voluntary position for twenty-five years, under every succeeding president, until his retirement in 1989. As chairman of the President's Committee on the Employment of People with Disabilities, Russell's job was to advise the White House on all legislative and policy issues related to disability, and to report annually to the president on the activities of the Committee. These issues included education, employment, transportation, barrier removal, healthcare, and advocacy. For forty-two years, Harold survived on the committee by remaining officially apolitical and unconditionally supportive of every president. He and several prominent veterans supported Harry Truman when General

MacArthur was relieved from duty. Truman was grateful. Amidst a firestorm of protest, Russell supported President Kennedy when the purview of the President's Committee was extended to include persons with mental illness and mental retardation. Kennedy was grateful. Some presidents afforded him greater access than others, some were more firmly committed to disability issues than others, but Harold Russell had kind words for each of them. Each was, after all, his commander in chief.

Other critical incidents, of a personal nature, served to endear some presidents to Harold more than others. Shortly after World War II, more than a dozen chartered veterans' organizations were determined to repossess a German-owned factory in New Jersey, and to redirect its $15-million-per-year profits toward the underwriting of their collective expenses. After refining their plan, they directly petitioned President Truman for the necessary authorization. "Gentlemen," said Truman, "this is classic veteran's grab, plain as day. I am against it, and I will not support it. Thank you for coming." Truman could have easily disguised his opposition and deferred the matter to a study group for later rejection. But his honesty and prompt decisiveness won the respect and admiration of everyone in attendance, including Harold Russell.

Some years later, Russell was charged with driving Senators Joe McCarthy and John F. Kennedy from O'Hare Field to downtown Chicago for a national AMVETS convention. A verbal debate ensued over a particular housing issue, and then deteriorated into a fist fight between the two, until Russell intervened with some unsolicited, benign, but timely information about convention logistics.

Harold recalls with regret the few missed opportunities for the President's Committee to have been elevated to new heights. One, in particular, has special relevance for him. In November 1963, President Kennedy returned from a visit to Germany, a high watermark in his presidency. During his visit, he observed remarkable advances in the use of prosthetics and orthotics. He summoned Harold Russell, and the two discussed the matter. Kennedy was uncomfortable that the U.S. was not the world leader in these technological developments. He asked Harold to chair a special commission to study the matter — a commission they would form together when he returned from his next trip. His next trip was to Dallas. The president never returned alive.

Harold also had his share of difficult interactions with the White House. When Massachusetts was the only state which Richard Nixon did not carry in the 1972 election, he set out to replace Harold Russell. He discussed plans for Harold's removal with Bob Haldemann. Fortunately, President Nixon became too distracted by Watergate to execute this and many other aspects of his domestic agenda. On another occasion, Harold Russell was in a reception line at the White House, where he extended his right hook in a greeting to Barbara Bush. "What am I supposed to do with that?" she quipped. "Well, most people shake it," he replied.

Not surprisingly, Harold Russell was personally inspired by President Roosevelt, although he regretted that Roosevelt took such extreme measures to mask his disability. Like most leaders in the disability community, Harold feels strongly that the new monument to Roosevelt should depict him in a wheelchair. He believes that Roosevelt's accomplishments and reputation are enhanced by the chair, that it adds to his image of leadership.

As a military man and politician, Harold greatly admired President Eisenhower, who initiated national efforts to create a barrier-free America for people with disabilities. However, of all the presidents under whom he served, Russell most admired President Truman, for his personal integrity. John F. Kennedy was a close second, in large part due to his Massachusetts roots, but also because of his sensitivity toward disability issues. He also had a natural rapport with Ronald Reagan, former director of the Screen Actors Guild, who spoke out strongly against McCarthyism. "He was not a president, but a king; although I am not sure that Nancy didn't run the country," he laughed. Harold Russell predicted a bright political future for Bill Clinton, due largely to his ability to learn from his mistakes. Noting the precise date, January 4, 1995, Russell confidently predicted the re-election of the "Truman-esque" Bill Clinton. He thought Clinton was a bright leader with a presidential "look." An astute observer of evolutionary politics, Russell also believes that the development of a viable, third political party is inevitable.

Having served under nine presidents, from Truman through Bush, Harold Russell perceived the job of president as the toughest, most thankless, no-win position in the world. The scrutiny of the modern press, and the sheer amount of information which one has to master, make the presidency a virtually impossible undertaking. Harold Russell is skeptical of everyone who seeks the job. He feels that we may never have a popular president again, and that transferable skills may be useful in rehabilitation, but are bad for the presidency. Those whose backgrounds are not political, such as Colin Powell or Ross Perot, are inherently unqualified. According to Harold, Perot was a "good merchant, but was vastly overrated, and out in left field, with respect to how government works...a very strange individual who could only have been created in America."

Harold believes Oliver North was an opportunist, a fake, an embarrassment to the uniform, and a criminal. He was a particularly dangerous individual who underscored for Harold Russell the dangers of extremism. Harold had seen Joe McCarthy at work, damaging careers and people themselves — many of them his Hollywood colleagues — with innuendo, inference, fear, and empty accusations. Harold Russell was openly scornful of "think-like-me" politics and of political correctness.

The advocacy career

Harold Russell had no regrets about forgoing an acting career to pursue an advocacy career in Washington, D.C. Russell asserts with amusement that, "there are more and better actors, directors, speakers, and connivers in D.C. than anywhere in the world; they are the real pros." Under the auspices of

Harold Russell Associates, Harold supported his family, primarily as a motivational speaker. Harold Russell's travels have taken him to every continent. He estimates that he has traveled the world approximately seven times, always providing humorous and inspirational messages about how we each can achieve more by maximizing our abilities. He also has consulted widely on the placement of people in industry and government. Harold founded the Harold Russell Motivational Institute, an organization which has enhanced the independence of people with disabilities by developing a national network of peer advisors.

In his travels, Harold Russell was determined to have fun along the way. Along with his second wife, Betty, and her brother, Matty, one or more of his lifelong companions often accompanied the Russells. These friends included Stan Allen, a publisher; Harold Keats, a builder; and Hugh Wiel, a federal judge. There are many stories about their revelry and practical jokes. Harold once poured ice water on Stan Allen, who was in an amorous position with a lady friend. In retribution, Stan locked Harold out in the hallway of the hotel — hookless and naked. On another occasion, Harold was in the men's room at O'Hare Field. He was struggling unsuccessfully with a stubborn zipper. The hooks would not cooperate that day. He requested help from Matty, who became so frustrated that his efforts took him to his knees — much to the bewilderment of some of the airport's passengers.

Throughout his life, Harold Russell has remained active in veterans- and disability-related organizations. With seed money of $5 million per year from the CIA, Harold helped organize veterans from 58 countries into the World Veterans Federation. In part, this move was intended to shore up relationships and communications among free world leaders. There was also the purpose of providing a mechanism to informally monitor the intentions of the communist military. Curiously, the organization was deemed a communist threat during the McCarthy hearings. As recently as 1994, in France, Harold Russell has participated in general assembly meetings focusing on rehabilitation efforts.

Later, Harold Russell served for many years as vice president of the World Veterans Fund. Harold also served three terms as national commander of AMVETS. He was chairman of the Massachusetts Industrial Accident Rehabilitation Board, and he served on the boards of the National Organization of Disability, People-to-People Committee for the Handicapped, and the national Challenge Committee on Disability. These were not armchair activities. At the age of eighty, Harold Russell visited veteran's hospitals in Central America. While there, he encountered American soldiers (advisers), for whom he placed phone calls of greeting and comfort upon returning home.

Harold Russell has been featured on every major TV news program and in every national publication in the country, including NBC's *Today Show*, ABC's *Good Morning America*, the *New York Times*, and the *Washington Post*. He has received scores of awards and citations, including honorary degrees from LaSalle University and the University of Massachusetts. He received the American Legion Citation of Meritorious Service in 1990, and in 1960, his star was placed on the Hollywood Walk of Fame.

Rita and the children

Harold had pursued Rita Russell since grammar school. His competition included Johnny Macpherson, Richard Nixon, and others — all handsome, dashing, and witty. He did not give himself much of a chance, but his mentor, Uncle Wolf (Wilfred Croucher) schooled him in the art of courtship, dancing, and romance. Coupled with his close friendship with Charley, Rita's brother, Uncle Wolf's coaching provided Harold with just enough of an edge to secure a commitment from Rita to be his prom date. At the dance, his cursory knowledge of only the fox-trot served him poorly when it came time to doing a waltz, tango, or rumba. But Harold knew no better; he persevered, and the couple plowed through every dance until the musicians went home. Harold felt like the kid next door, like her kid brother's best pal, but hardly like the dynamic and charming hero that he longed to be for Rita — his best and only girl.

For the remainder of his teen years and well into his twenties, Rita was there — consistent, lovely, and ever-popular. But he had to contend with Nixon and Macpherson, and other suitors, as well. Harold felt that if he could become more established, get higher pay, more security in the grocery store or in some other business — if he could only be somebody — then maybe he could muster the courage to ask for Rita's hand. Indeed, she was a lovely girl, but Harold's hesitation cost him. Richard Nixon, now a local policeman — handsome and brave in his uniform — cut in on him: Rita and Richard were married in June of 1941.

The marriage was tumultuous from the beginning. It yielded one child, Gerald, and considerable domestic unrest. When the two got divorced in the summer of 1942, Harold, the soldier, and Rita began dating again. Throughout his military career, Harold and Rita exchanged letters and visited on furloughs, and the romance blossomed. They frequently discussed marriage and the need for Gerald to have a father. Harold felt it was best to defer plans of marriage until he returned safe and unharmed from his overseas duty.

During the period of recovery from his injuries, Harold was in turmoil regarding their future. Characteristic of his own psychological adjustment to his disabilities, he regularly insisted that the couple break up, convinced that Rita would be better off with a "whole man." Through it all, she was steadfast. The story of their relationship, its ups and downs, and gradual improvement, served to mirror his own awareness and acceptance of his disabilities.

At last, Harold's dream of marriage to Rita was about to be realized. He and Rita were married in 1946, during the shooting of *The Best Years of Our Lives*. Harold was determined to raise Gerald as his own son. A year later, they added a daughter, Adelle. As the years passed, Rita and Adelle became nearly consumed with the subject and practice of horse jumping. The two awakened Harold at 6:00 A.M. on Saturdays for horse shows, which Harold loathed because he hated the smell. Nonetheless, from May to September, he drove the two to the shows, although he often slept in the car during their performances. Harold has remained close to his daughter. In her late forties, Adelle is divorced with two children: Tommy, a teacher in Albuquerque, and Jennifer, a veterinarian who shares Adelle's passion for horses.

Rita was the antithesis of Harold Russell. Shy, timid, and insecure, Rita preferred the life of a homemaker to Harold's passion for adventure and travel. She hated flying, which was a passion for Harold. She would not accompany Harold to the Academy Awards, so he attended with his brother, Les, in tow. Rita often expressed that she felt inferior to the politicians and celebrities with whom Harold associated. Her great love was Adelle and their cherished horse jumping. She was a chain smoker, and a more-than-occasional drinker — "for confidence." Harold loved and respected Rita, but they were very different. In 1972, after twenty-six years of marriage, living in both Whalen and Framingham, Massachusetts, Rita died suddenly of a heart attack.

Gerald assumed the name Gerry Russell shortly after his adoption by Harold. He was a daredevil as a youth, a stress seeker who loved excitement. He once "borrowed" Harold's Cadillac and drove it at sixty mph, long before the age at which permits were allowed. Gerry graduated from the University of New Hampshire with a psychology degree. He then found all the excitement he could manage as an Air Force captain in Vietnam, where he earned two commendations for bravery, including one for landing a burning airplane. Gerry married his childhood sweetheart and the couple had two daughters. After dabbling in construction, Gerry became established in Florida as a commercial pilot for Eastern Airlines. Still, he was never quite the same after Vietnam.

Much to his dismay, Harold's relationship with Gerry just never seemed to "click." Harold, who had worked hard for everything he had, was constantly perturbed by what he saw as his son's sense of entitlement. Gerry's relationship with his wife became strained, and in spite of Harold's repeated trips to dissuade the couple from breaking up, the couple was divorced in 1980. Fourteen-year-old Debbie resided with her mother while sixteen-year-old Wendy continued to live with Gerry in Miami. It was at this time that Gerry accelerated a three-year involvement with Kathi Anderson, a married flight attendant recently separated from her husband, Lance.

Theirs was the story of a love triangle, and of sudden death. Gerald Russell, thirty-nine, and Lance Anderson, forty-two, were hardly friends; in fact, they hardly knew one another. Ironically, both were native New Englanders. Both loved to fly. Both were pilots for Eastern Airlines. And both were in love with the same thirty-nine-year-old flight attendant, Kathi. Kathi was torn between the two men and was unable to choose. She had recently reconciled with Lance, whose business interests were beginning to soar. Gerry became increasingly obsessed with Kathi. Excessive drinking and bizarre behavior ensued, including multiple speeding violations. Even though she had reconciled with Lance, Kathi openly dated Gerry during this period in situations that included her seven-year-old daughter, Lisa. Lance hired a private detective to monitor Gerry's relationship with Kathi and acquired a total of four handguns, three of which mysteriously disappeared over a period of a few weeks.

On February 24, 1982, from 7 P.M. to 9 P.M., Gerry played tennis and had a few drinks in Coral Gables. He returned to his Miami home to watch television with Wendy, and his drinking continued. At about 11 P.M., Gerry took a phone call from Kathi. She told him that Lance had a gun and was coming home to attack her. Gerry drove off in a rush, leaving the television on and the garden hose running. Only Kathi and Gerry know the truth about precisely what happened next. What is known is that Lance and a business associate, Frank Armstrong, pulled up to the Anderson home in the Redlands section of south Dade county. Gerry, clad in a jogging suit and ski mask, fired a gun several times, from a distance of three feet. Lance was struck once in the shoulder and twice in the face — he was killed at the wheel of his new Mercedes. Lance managed to fire a single shot from his derringer, hitting Gerry in the chest. Armstrong's shoulder was grazed by a bullet, but he escaped to his office in another building on the property, where he armed himself with his own gun and sat waiting in the dark, terrified.

Neighbors summoned the police. The murder weapon, an Arminiums Titan revolver, was found near the fence. It was later confirmed to be one of Lance's missing handguns. Six minutes after the slaying, a wounded Gerry Russell was found unconscious and slumped over the steering wheel of his pickup truck, which had slammed into a pole less than a mile from the murder scene. Cool, calm, and unruffled in her formal statement to the police, Kathi identified Gerry Russell as the assailant. She stated that she loved Lance and had told Gerry that she was not going to leave her husband.

Gerry Russell underwent surgery for his wound. Five months later, an emotional trial ensued in a Dade County Circuit Court. There was not an empty seat in the gallery. The question was whether the killing was premeditated. Pleading insanity, Gerry's defense attorney Joel Hirschhorn directed the jury's attention to Kathi Anderson, who "...gave him [Russell] the gun...and manipulated him into his state of mind. Kathi Anderson *managed* Gerry Russell...she hated Lance Anderson, but she loved his money...she belongs in that empty chair beside my client." The first jury ballot was seven to four to convict — for second-degree murder. After more than six hours of often-loud and angry deliberation, the Dade County Circuit Court jury convicted Gerald Russell of first-degree murder in the slaying of Lance Anderson, but acquitted him of attempted first-degree murder in the shooting of Frank Armstrong. Judge Joseph P. Farina imposed the mandatory sentence of life imprisonment, with a twenty-five-year term before parole consideration.

Kathi Anderson would not submit to a polygraph. She inherited a considerable estate, estimated at $1.5 million. In the months that followed, Lance's parents requested an independent executor of the estate, claiming,

"We do not feel she [Kathi] is suitable, nor qualified, for this post." Their reasons included her lack of business experience, and their perception that "there is a cloud on this case."

In an unsuccessful attempt to have the charges reduced, Harold contributed to Gerald's defense every dollar he could manage, in excess of $10,000. To this day, Harold's relationship with Gerald and his granddaughters remains strained. They believe Harold could have provided the personal and political intercession necessary to have Gerald's sentence commuted. Harold did not, and these events troubled him for years to come. Harold wanted to understand his son, and the others who had served in Vietnam. Harold's and their war experiences, and subsequent personal histories, had been so very different.

Crossed hooks and fixed bayonets

In his research of the Vietnam war, Harold discovered a curious and uncomfortable statistic — approximately 250,000 veterans comprised one-third of the entire homeless population in America. A full 60% of these were Vietnam veterans. As he continued his self-education, he discovered that many homeless Vietnam veterans shared several common characteristics, including a lack of work skills that could be easily transferred to the civilian world. There were also unaffordable housing, chemical dependency, post-traumatic stress syndrome, and other problems. Men and women who once rose to the call of duty with "fixed bayonets" had found themselves in poverty, fighting a battle for survival on the streets. This became Harold Russell's calling in his later years. Their voices reached out to him.

When Ken Smith, executive director of The Project to Shelter Homeless Veterans, discovered Harold's restless transition into retirement in nearby Hyannis, he dropped everything and drove to the Cape to pay a visit. Harold was interested in Ken's work and probed him for more specifics. Ken told Harold that most homeless veterans had been homeless for less than a year. The New England Shelter for Homeless Veterans in Boston was successfully placing more than 85% of its clients in jobs, permanent housing, or both. Homeless veterans were once again becoming productive citizens, responsible parents, and taxpayers.

It was time for Harold to travel to Boston to take a look at the project first-hand. The dreary weather and aggravating traffic, in a thriving city with an inadequate infrastructure, established the bleak mood. The project to shelter homeless veterans was located at 17 Court Street in Boston's financial district, directly across from the state house and city hall. The structure itself was imposing — ten stories, 140,000 square feet — a brick-and-mortar testament to the interaction of asbestos and years of neglect. The abandoned (and nearly condemned) federal building had been formerly occupied by the Department of Veterans Affairs. In 1989, a creative lease was arranged under the McKinney Homeless Act, which provides surplus government property to not-for-profit organizations serving the homeless. The clever acquisition of this property was one of several remarkable acts of advocacy by an equally remarkable leader.

Ken Smith had sounded the charge. In an effort to better understand homelessness, and perhaps to understand Gerald, Harold Russell responded to the call. The alleviation of homelessness among all U.S. veterans was a cause to which Harold became deeply committed. Though he was approaching eighty years of age, Harold Russell became co-chairman of the project and ventured into Boston weekly to provide wisdom, experience, counsel, guidance, intercession, and networking assistance to project managers. More valued still was the inspiration and encouragement he gave to the clients — whether they had served in the Army, Navy, Marines, Air Force, Coast Guard, or Reserves, or in World War I, World War II, Korea, Vietnam, Panama, Grenada, the Persian Gulf, Somalia, Haiti, or Bosnia. The simple act of his presence among them had a therapeutic effect which human service professionals envied. Ken Smith knew this, and exploited it to the hilt, in order to prevail in a domestic and social struggle that he viewed as an ongoing extension of the war itself. The war was not over for Ken Smith.

In its brief history, the project has served over 9,000 veterans from all fifty states and six territories. It currently serves nearly 30,000 meals per week. There are 130 staff members, including psychologists, social workers, job-training instructors, and financial-assistance counselors. In its classrooms, veterans are trained as bus drivers, security guards, line cooks, and computer repairmen. There are programs for housing, medical care, legal assistance, literacy training, mental health, financial management, substance abuse treatment, post-traumatic stress disorder, and Agent Orange assistance. Within this military-like structure, the themes of sobriety and self-help permeate all levels of care along the continuum: crisis intervention (the "cot squad"), emergency shelter, transitional housing, permanent housing, and day programming.

When all is said and done, there are four striking features of the embryonic project which account for its effectiveness. First, is the insistence by management on abstinence from drugs and alcohol on the parts of all clients. Second, there is a strong employment focus, which includes four on-site training programs, in occupations that are high in demand and pay a livable wage. Third, the military decorum enhances camaraderie, minimizes insecurities associated with street life, and provides all clients and staff a common language, culture, and set of ground rules. Finally, and probably most importantly, there is the zealousness, commitment, and leadership of Ken Smith.

The handsome, charismatic Vietnam veteran is considered by many to be a living paradox. A self-proclaimed agnostic, Smith makes repeated references to his Catholic upbringing. Smith is a professional persuader who describes himself as "not sick, but angry." Formerly in the printing business, Ken Smith visited "the Wall" in 1986. This is a gripping experience for all who visit, but powerful beyond words for those who served in Vietnam. In his attentive manner, he noticed a large number of veterans, same-age peers who were meandering about in Washington Park. In casual conversation, he made inquiries as to where each one lived, what each called "home." The response was consistent: "Here, the park." Since that moment, Ken Smith has been nothing less than obsessed with bringing each veteran "all the way home." What resulted was a new, 1990s campaign in an old, but incomplete, war. This was very different from other Vietnam war-era campaigns. This one would not be lost.

There are few people less popular than a bona fide crusader, but Ken Smith is precisely that. He describes homelessness as a disability, and enumerates its many handicapping effects. Smith's own hypomania and polyphasic thinking are readily apparent to visitors. Ideas burst forth as he alternately sits, stands, paces, and brandishes his bayonet — which he periodically swings and stabs into an otherwise impressive conference table.

Ken Smith is outspoken, brash, obnoxious, demanding, petulant, and angry; yet he is also literate, dynamic, articulate, intense, and engaging. At their first meeting, Harold Russell found Ken Smith to be as bewildering, tumultuous, chaotic, and multi-directional as Vietnam itself. "Fixed bayonets..." is the project slogan. Ken Smith does not hesitate to assemble his "color guard" in full-dress uniform for an immediate, vocal, and public demonstration against all who oppose, or are perceived to impede, the realization of his goal: the immediate eradication of homelessness for all veterans of the U.S. military. Without hesitation, apology, or embarrassment, Ken Smith will challenge what he perceives to be the benign neglect of seemingly every individual he encounters in his anything-but-routine daily life. He deliberately creates an atmosphere of dissonance and discomfort to cause the listener to focus on his message.

Some of his efforts have been more targeted. He once approached the Kuwaiti embassy in Washington, demanding that he be given ownership of a particular kind of oil, in order to be able to fund the project for veterans of the Gulf War. He crashed numerous receptions of V.A. officials demanding an answer to his question: How could 250,000 homeless veterans be ignored in the $40-billion-per-year budget of the Department of Veterans Affairs? He made a formal appeal to the state department that 5% of all foreign aid be diverted to the resolution of the dilemma of homeless veterans, reminding the secretary of state that "charity begins at home." Under the same rubric, he vehemently objected to the release of $60 million to relocate Russian soldiers from Berlin as a part of the liberation of Eastern Europe.

This style of advocacy was foreign to Harold Russell, who had always had similar goals but had relied on non-violence, patience, tact, diplomacy, protocol, and his well-honed skills of communication and negotiation. Harold admired Ken Smith, however — especially his love for his Vietnam brothers. Observing them together, one appreciates the uniqueness of the veteran's status when it comes to the design and administration of their rehabilitation programs. There are bonds among the clients that relate to common fears, a common experience, and a code of honor — bonds that must be acknowledged. Harold Russell understood this well. Yet Harold was bewildered by Ken Smith and his methods. Is it conceivable that some of Ken Smith's advocacy tactics may have enhanced Harold's own effectiveness with the President's Committee? From his association with Ken Smith, Harold Russell acquired a deeper understanding of the special circumstances surrounding the war in Vietnam, which affected the lives of all who had served there, mostly for the worst. Harold expressed regret that his understanding was somewhat belated.

On more than one occasion, Harold stepped in to temper the strategic plans of the aggressive executive director. On an equal number of occasions, he participated in the "mopping up" of some ill-timed or politically bankrupt maneuvers. Said Smith, "When Harold crosses those hooks, it's time to shut up and listen." (Smith fully expects to mount the hooks on his office wall after Harold's passing, as a salute to his contributions to the struggle). Says Smith:

> Harold Russell is an American icon. As a tactician and diplomat, he has done more for veterans worldwide than any man alive. Me? I am like a raptor, I prefer a full frontal assault.

Harold Russell used his celebrity to contact other famous individuals when influence or financial assistance was necessary. Ken Smith describes Harold Russell as the military equivalent of "Frank Sinatra and Enrico Caruso combined," and himself as Snoop-Doggy-Dog. The mix is not one of oil and water, since both men share an appreciation for the music: an understanding of a common problem and solution. Only their styles differ. Moreover, their mutual respect is readily apparent to the observer. In reference to Harold Russell, Ken Smith describes himself as "...sitting at the right hook of the father."

In spite of his role with the project and other self-education efforts, Harold Russell still struggles in his attempt to understand the Vietnam war.

> To this day, I am unable to figure out why we were fighting there. I could never disagree with the conscientious objectors. However, I did object to those who deserted after being sworn into service. Vietnam was the most tragic war ever fought. It was a wrong war in a wrong place. There is one thing about Vietnam I have come to understand clearly — the Vietnam veteran got fucked.

Harold Russell does not completely understand Vietnam, but he does understand loss. He has experienced the premature, abrupt, and tragic losses of a father, wife, and son. Call it compensation, restitution, a second chance, or redemption. Harold Russell would not allow this son, nor his cause, to fail.

Betty and the very best years

There are few places as pleasant as Cape Cod in May. Harold Russell's friend, Uncle Jack Croucher, a retired writer for Associated Press, was now minding Angelo's Grocery Store in Needham. He hadn't tried his hand at matchmaking in some time, but he thought there was romance in the air. The combination made sense, but maybe it was too obvious. Betty had been a dedicated employee at Angelo's since she moved to the Cape. Word had it that she had been an even better nurse for fifteen years. Divorced for twenty-three years, Betty was the mother of four and the grandmother of seven. She was so attractive, it was hard to believe she was still single. Harold had been widowed for nine years now, and Jack thought he needed looking after. What was there to lose? A blind date was set. Harold went to the Cape and escorted Betty to the Paddock Restaurant.

Something clicked; something must have, because Harold went to the Cape every weekend after that. He called Betty every night. Was it their immediate compatibility, the spring air, the spontaneity of a trip to California, Harold's good nature, or Uncle Jack's good judgment? Whatever the inspiration, the two were married less than three months later, in August 1981.

Unlike Rita, Betty was fun-loving and adventurous. She loved to travel, and was unabashed in the presence of celebrity. Much to the surprise of Hollywood director Richard Donner, Betty once yelled "cut" during the shooting of *Inside Moves*, in order to towel off a sweating Harold Russell.

Their Cape Cod house is across from the Kennedy compound and one mile from the beach. It is a New England-style home and impeccably neat, with the exception of Harold's messy basement office, which seems to provide evidence of earthquake activity in Hyannis. They have ample time to read fiction and history. A visitor might find *The Decline and Fall of the Roman Empire* on the coffee table. Ably assisted by their cat, Tom, Betty provides love, companionship, advocacy, support, and more personal assistance than Harold requires.

The couple loves to travel. They have been to every continent, and scores of countries. If a stopover in Las Vegas can be arranged, that is all the better. Seven-card stud is more than a passing interest for Harold. A Native American casino in neighboring Connecticut is well worth the two-hour drive. On quiet days, he spends hours at the computer, playing poker or golf.

Opening and reading the mail from friends and admirers all over the world consumes a good part of the day. The couple was recently deliberating the origins of a greeting card from San Diego; they could not recall how they knew the sender, but a photograph of a newborn baby was enclosed. Harold said to Betty, "I don't remember them, and as for the baby, I didn't do it."

Betty's siblings, children, and grandchildren are regular visitors for conversation, cards, and pool playing. Their extended families get along famously. Betty's brother, Matthew, is a key player in their lives. A retired postal worker, World War II veteran, and recipient of the Silver Star, Matty provides keen competition for Harold at the pool table. Indeed, Harold is incessantly fawned over and even smothered in his retirement. His response? "Let's just say I'm not complaining."

Rounds two, three, and four with severe disability

Lightning does not strike in the same place twice — or so they say. But it did — and it struck a third time, then a fourth. In 1984, Harold Russell was going about his business in Washington, D.C. as chairman of the President's Committee on Employment of the Handicapped, when the pain began. Throughout the next day it worsened, and Betty, a former nurse, would wait no longer. The couple returned to Massachusetts General Hospital in Boston, where Betty browbeat the chief oncologist into admitting Harold into his personal care. Prostate cancer was diagnosed. Six lesions were detected in the spine, ribs, and hip. Harold was informed that with luck, estrogen, and radiation therapy, he might survive another two years.

The happy, productive couple would not accept a death sentence. They sought a second opinion at the Sloan Kettering Institute in New York, and a third opinion from the National Cancer Institute. The diagnosis and prognosis were confirmed, but Dr. DeVita added that positive research findings had been reported at Laval University Medical Center in Quebec, Canada. Betty called to schedule an evaluation, and was told that their waiting list was now at three months — minimum. Betty was not to be denied. Citing Harold's Canadian roots and brandishing credentials from the White House to the Academy of Motion Picture Arts and Sciences, Harold Russell was scheduled for evaluation five days later.

Dr. Fernand Labrie and Dr. Andre Dupont examined Harold Russell and found three more lesions in the groin, for a new total of nine lesions. By using a combination of drugs: oral flutamide and injectable LHRH (lutenizing hormone-releasing hormone), they sought to completely block the substance in the male hormone that feeds the prostate cancer. After two days, the couple returned home, where Harold took the pills and Betty administered the injections. Within ninety days, the nodule on the prostate had completely disappeared, and the other lesions were gone after a period of fifteen months. Harold Russell was in complete remission, and most men would be overwhelmed with joy.

But Harold Russell was troubled; were it not for his Canadian ancestry, celebrity status, insistent partner, and private resources, he would not have experienced the wonders of Laval University Medical Center. What about the other 80,000 American men who are diagnosed with prostate cancer each year? Flutamide was not FDA approved, so the medication regimen, at $5000 per month, was not reimbursable. But Harold Russell was cured, so why should he care?

Harold Russell did care, however. Prostate cancer was the leading cause of death in men over sixty. His research showed that flutamide was in widespread use in Switzerland, Germany, and even the Soviet Union. Harold and Betty used the influence they had in Washington and the lessons they had learned about the power of the mass media, to wage war on the FDA's excessively strict standards to protect public safety. The review process was accelerated, and flutamide achieved FDA approval in 1997, as an effective agent in the treatment of prostate cancer. Still, widespread endorsement of the new drug was gradual because, Harold believed, it obviated the need for more lucrative surgical procedures.

With age, Harold's health has deteriorated. Activities of daily living have become more difficult, and Betty has increased proportionately her levels of personal assistance. There have been occasional falls, broken bones, and complications from bronchitis and diabetes. Compliance with a diabetic diet is challenging, and has been a source of spirited debate between Harold and Betty. Although his affability and good nature continue, he finds it markedly more convenient, and effective, to deploy Betty to redress his grievances these days. To her irritation, Harold occasionally gets mad about something and tells Betty, "Now you call them up and give them hell." Apparently, Harold has become the good cop, Betty the bad. Instinctively, Harold knows when he has pushed matters too far; just in time, he will produce the right gift — flowers, jewelry, or a coat. Their romance continues.

Harold's health problems did not end with prostate cancer. In the fall of 1995, he stepped on a toothpick and later noticed a redness and soreness in his right foot. Doctors mistakenly diagnosed it as athlete's foot, but an infection brewed, leading to cellulitis. Eventually, after additional misdiagnoses, Harold became disoriented, confused, and agitated. Physicians determined that the foot was gangrenous. After a series of three surgeries, approximately one-third of his foot was amputated. The two-week hospitalization was followed by three weeks of inpatient rehabilitation, followed by outpatient and home-based therapies. Regaining mobility was complicated for Harold because assistive and adaptive devices had to be custom-made to work with his prosthetic arms. Expressions of support poured in, including those from President Clinton and Jesse Brown, secretary of the Department of Veterans Affairs, a favorite of Harold's.

Despite his progress, Harold was gradually becoming more dependent in his activities of daily living. With the assistance and support from Betty, Harold prevailed. He strove to remain as active as possible, and proclaimed himself the oldest triple amputee in the world. The couple managed another trip to Hollywood, where Harold was cast in a supporting role in *Dogtown*, a movie about the adventures of an aspiring young actor. Harold played a disabled veteran and owner of a cigar store in the movie's small town. The director, Mr. Higgenlooper, had seen *The Best Years of Our Lives* nine times and insisted on having Harold play the role. Harold reveled in the frequent opportunities to advise the young director, who often asked, "Do you think Wyler would have done it like that?"

In the fall of 1996, a new procedure was needed — this time a partial replacement of Harold's left hip. He faced more surgery, more rehabilitation, and nearly four weeks of hospitalization — more challenges for Harold, Betty, the therapists, and the designers of prosthetic and orthotic equipment.

Rehabilitation was becoming increasingly compromised by the combination of age and additional disabilities. A wheelchair had become necessary for traveling more than a few steps. Perhaps acutely sensing his mortality, Harold became impatient with all matters relating to his health and personal care. Betty was now stretched to the limit with her attendant-care duties.

What's all the fuss?

Harold Russell had been retired for three years. When he turned seventy-eight, it was clear to him that his prime earning years were over. In addition, he had had some unanticipated expenses, including cancer treatment in Canada, an eye operation for Betty, legal expenses for Gerald, and a septic-tank problem in his yard. The couple was far from destitute, but it would be nice to have some tangible cash security in their latter years. Besides, there was a planned Pacific vacation — a trip that included visits to Hong Kong, Thailand, and Singapore. The couple discussed their financial situation for nearly eight months before arriving at a decision, and now the time had come. On July 30, 1992, Harold took his Best Supporting Actor award, and placed it on an auction block in New York City. The auction was to be held on August 6.

The Academy of Motion Picture Arts and Sciences was furious. Its president, Karl Malden, sent a letter to Russell urging him to reconsider. It read, "These Oscars...should not become objects of mere commerce." Malden called Harold Russell, offering a $20,000 loan in exchange for the Oscar, which would be returned to Russell once the loan was paid. Russell refused.

The electronic and print media swarmed the neighborhood. At the modest Russell residence in Hyannis, reporters and TV cameramen lined up, and the phone rang nonstop. There were reporters from *People* magazine and *Entertainment Tonight*; correspondents arrived from Toronto, Germany, and London. The stories became increasingly exaggerated, reporting that the couple had no money for a needed eye operation for Betty. In truth, a simple cataract operation had been scheduled. The story blossomed when it was learned that other Russell memorabilia would be included in the auction — letters from presidents, and autographed photos of Babe Ruth, Samuel Goldwyn, Frederic March, and Dana Andrews.

The critics raged on. Russell responded that he had been paid less than $10,000 for his part in a picture which had grossed tens of millions of dollars. If the Oscar was not an object of commerce, why had Malden suggested a collateral value of $20,000? He repeated that he simply wanted the security that the extra money would bring — a cushion, of sorts. After all, he could not take the Oscar with him to the next life. An understanding of Harold's decision came slowly to those who had not experienced his upbringing during the Depression; for many it would not come at all.

On August 6, 1992, the Oscar sold for $60,500. This was the first time an Academy Award had been sold by its winner. Since 1950, recipients of Academy Awards have been required to sign legal papers promising never to sell their Oscars, but this rule followed Harold's 1946 award. John Lennon won an Oscar in 1971 for the Best Original Song for the movie, *Let It Be*. In 1976, he donated his Oscar to the Southbury Training School (for disabled children) in Connecticut, which auctioned it for $600. Observing the success of Harold Russell's auction, the new owner auctioned Lennon's Oscar in 1992 — for $100,000!

Harold Russell has given serious consideration to initiating a lawsuit to recover more revenues for his contribution to *The Best Years of Our Lives*. The paltry $10,000 paid to him by contract seems inadequate by today's standards, especially since the movie has made millions on network and cable television, video sales, and in international distribution. None of these distribution mechanisms, nor the windfall profits that would result, were even considered when the contract was signed in 1946. Who could have ever known?

Life lessons

Even in his eighties, Harold Russell gives much more thought to living than to dying. Nonetheless, the latter subject has been considered. He recalls an old expression from his military days: "It is important to leave the camp a cleaner and better place than you found it." This is what he wishes for himself; that the world will be a somewhat better place for his experience in it, particularly for veterans and people with disabilities. There are many lessons he has learned, which he hopes will be remembered long after he is gone. These are among Harold's very special pearls of wisdom:

On advocacy

"Effective advocacy need not be exclusively adversarial in character. There is a time and a place for diplomacy, tact, and patience. For employers and policy makers, there are many competing concerns, and their priorities must be respected. Militancy has its place, and it certainly looks glamorous, but it is marginally effective with employers and politicians. I have always preferred the use of carrots.

On balance, the Americans with Disabilities Act is terrific because it makes people pay attention to important issues. However, the employer mandates may do more harm than good. It is against human nature to tell people they *have* to do something, especially in America.

To increase labor force participation among persons with disabilities, employers and their needs must be considered. In my day, this meant advocacy and education with Fortune 500 companies. The focus must shift now from large to smaller employers, because that is where hiring will occur in the century ahead. Contemporary advocates think that laws can be passed to bully and intimidate employers. They are wrong.

Local advocacy is most effective. As responsibilities and resources shift to the states, education and advocacy efforts must be localized. For example, the development and empowerment of the Governors' Committees on the Employment of People with Disabilities has been the single biggest contribution of the President's Committee.

Equal attention must be paid to public access and employment issues. The two go hand in hand. Advancements cannot be made in one area without the other. This lesson has come late to me, but it is not too late to be helpful in moving forward. Particularly impressive are the recent gains in improving access to sports and recreation, like the Special Olympics and the Paralympics. Access to computers and new technologies is equally important. These investments will pay big dividends.

Some disabilities are not more legitimate than others. All consumer groups should be organized and focus upon the realization of common goals. They can work with other strong groups such as older Americans, who have more disabilities themselves. The advantages, privileges, effective strategies, and tactics possessed by select groups must be shared. For example, until President Kennedy, the President's Committee was for physically disabled persons only. Against much resistance, the president insisted on a change in name and mission, and he was correct.

If one becomes disabled in the performance of a public service, that individual has a special status. This status can be adaptive and should be explicitly addressed in the course of rehabilitation. Similarly, most veterans have difficulty transferring military skills into the civilian workforce. In a time of declining support for vocational training, the unique needs of the veteran should be remembered."

On rehabilitation

"Rehabilitation outcome has more to do with psychological than medical processes. In order to be effective, clients must be challenged. Such challenges are most effective when extended by successful rehabilitants. This is what Charley McGonegal did for me. More involvement by disabled persons is desirable, but the contributions of non-disabled rehabilitationists cannot be discounted.

Disability does not occur as a retribution for evil. I once thought that perhaps my injuries were a punishment of sorts for what I perceived to be a number of earlier failures — academic, social, and career. Such a position is not only inaccurate, it is an enormous impediment to rehabilitation.

There is no substitute for the love and support of one person throughout the rehabilitation experience, especially to help manage the psychological issues. Rita was there for me the first time; Betty the second time and beyond. For people who are married when they become severely disabled, the divorce rate is very high. People should take their vows seriously. 'For better or for worse' means just that.

Discovering and emphasizing residual capabilities, particularly as these relate to employment and performing activities of daily living, are the essence of rehabilitation. Real adjustment for me began when I realized that it is not what you've lost that counts, but what you have left. I was injured on D-Day. It was my own private D-Day. I had to set up a beachhead on reality.

Rehabilitation should be a realistic and practical endeavor. It should emphasize function over form. For me this was illustrated by my original preference for cosmetic, but useless, prosthetic hands, vs. functional, though less-attractive hooks. Similarly, I had to face the reality of my own situation, and the responsibility for making adjustments was on me, not on my mother, Rita, nor on my friends. I began to stop regarding myself as a freak. I began to discover that my disability was nothing to be ashamed of. If I behaved in a manner that conveyed acceptance and comfort, others would become more comfortable and the discussion would soon focus on something other than my impairment.

Rehabilitation should be a highly individualized endeavor. Disabled persons should be encouraged to relearn functional activities in a manner that they find comfortable and easy; to find the road that suits them best. There is no universal road to recovery that should, or could, be followed by all.

Rehabilitation hospitals are extremely valuable. People like Howard Rusk and Henry Kessler were great innovators. The personnel and services are extraordinary. But the process of disengagement from the hospital is very frightening. Hospitalization provides a moratorium on expectations, and it is easy to slip into disability as a career, even as a lifestyle. Moving patients from the hospital to the community should occur as quickly as possible, but transitional steps should be provided to make re-entry a more gradual process.

Among the most difficult things to learn in rehabilitation is the ability to ask for and accept assistance. At one point, I had mastered nearly all activities of daily living except tying my tie. I asked Charley McGonegal how he managed this. 'Marry your girlfriend,' he said, 'and she'll fix your tie for you.'

The single, most valuable role of government in rehabilitation is the support of training and education programs. These can equip people with disabilities with specialized skills for which there is a measurable demand in the world of work, today and for the foreseeable future. A G.I. Bill of Rights for the Disabled is needed, similar to what veterans enjoyed after World War II. This would give people with disabilities direct financial support to attend regular colleges, universities, and vocational-technical schools. Education is still the great equalizer.

The state-federal vocational rehabilitation program has an excellent design. The lack of effectiveness is best explained by the reality that most state directors are politicians and bureaucrats, not disabled individuals or rehabilitation professionals. 'If you want your car fixed, would you take it to a politician?' Ed Roberts is an example of the ideal program manager.

What Americans know about disability and rehabilitation is a valuable commodity. It should be exported internationally to help improve the overall human condition. Exchanges of experts and technology can serve to improve strained relationships with other countries and help to secure the peace."

Important values

"Mine has been a life characterized by opportunity and luck. On many, many occasions I was just in the right place at the right time. But one has to position him/herself to take advantage of these, and this is only achieved by maintaining optimism, building relationships, and incessant hard work. My disabling injuries and illnesses are far from the most important or defining moments of my life.

A positive aspect of military life, the rehabilitation experience, and movie making was the camaraderie. All artificial differences regarding class, religion, race, nationality, politics, social positions, and the like would disappear in the aggressive pursuit of a common enterprise. Most of our wars have been fought to protect our rights to have different ideas. Not necessarily to accept them, but to concede their right to be heard. In the absence of a common goal, intolerance and second-class citizenship seem to emerge. The price of liberty has been too great to abide this. In the hundreds of speeches I have made under the sponsorship of veterans organizations, civic groups, movie studios, rehabilitation associations, or the President's Committee, my consistent message has been to promote tolerance and full citizenship for all Americans."

On seven-card stud

"The cards are dealt, two down and one up. If your two hole cards are not as good as anything you see on the table, get out immediately."

chapter two

Evan Kemp

Al Condeluci

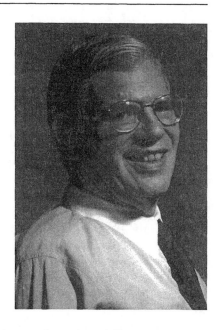

Introduction

It was 1954, and a bright, somewhat sensitive twelve-year-old boy was sitting in the living room, reading. With the cold Cleveland wind blowing outside, the boy's mother and dad were in the next room struggling with the news they had just received. Their son, the light of their lives, had ALS, the dreaded amyotrophic lateral sclerosis, Lou Gehrig's disease. They had been told he might live for only two more years. For the past four years or so, he had been weak, falling down, and having difficulty with his strength. Mom knew immediately that something was wrong. Dad had been more optimistic. Now their worst fears were confirmed. What should they do? How could they tell their son? Should he have to bear the weight of this tragic news?

It was 1963, a glorious day in central Virginia. The leaves were ablaze and the University of Virginia campus was even more beautiful than its catalog brochure boasted. A third-year law student, that same Cleveland lad, was making his way back to his dorm from the myriad interviews routinely held for the graduating law students. He was convinced that he would be quickly recruited for a major law firm. After all, he had excellent grades, was active on campus, and was now ready to make his mark in the world.

1-57444-083-7/00/$0.00+$.50

But the response to his interviews fell far short of the mark. His struggle with strength and endurance and his constant falling had cast a long shadow over his dreams. After all was said and done, the thirty-nine faces on the other side of the interview desk told the story: this young man lacked the stamina to make it in a large law firm. It would be better for him to consider a lesser role in law. This, he was told, would be best. Under the weight of this experience, the young man was moving slower than usual. His dream was being put on hold.

It was 1971, and the swiftness of the accident made it unavoidable. Later, in his mind, the young Securities and Exchange Commission lawyer would see the garage door sweep down on him in hauntingly slow motion. Yet there was nothing he could do, and before he knew it, he was knocked to the ground, caught in the pain of a broken leg. The net result was the permanent need for a wheelchair. Interestingly enough, Evan Kemp, years before, had asked for a wheelchair to help deal with his constant falls, the embarrassment, and the unpredictability of his situation. But his parents and doctors had advised against it. They told him that if he became accustomed to a wheelchair, the world would treat him differently; he would be seen as a lesser man. The young man was not so sure but followed the advice of his family. Now the wheelchair was a reality, but he was determined it would not get in his way. He would succeed with his wit, intelligence, and hard work. Two years later, this same attorney filed a discrimination suit against the Securities and Exchange Commission. It seemed that the SEC felt that a man who used a wheelchair did not have the capacity to supervise two staff members.

These are but a few of the many experiences that have unfolded in the life and times of Evan Kemp, Jr., and in 1995, on a warm fall day in the shadows of his study, he looked back on his life and career in the first of a series of interviews.

Evan Kemp is a soft-spoken man, with strong, inquisitive eyes. Although he is graying, his face and appearance belie his sixty years of age. Using a raised wheelchair, slightly tilted back, he speaks in an easy and deliberate manner, choosing his words carefully, being quick to clarify or accentuate a point.

For some thirty years now, Evan Kemp has been a leader in the disability movement, but his has been a different route than that of most other advocates. A self-proclaimed economic conservative, and now a loyal Republican, Evan has often been on the other side of disability issues from most of his peers. He has rejected the "take it to the streets" approach of advocacy and has preferred to explore the individual rights/empowerment piece of the puzzle. More than most, he has used the power of the pen to promote his ideas and ideals. He aligned himself with conservative thinkers well before it became fashionable to promote disability issues. As his public activity has given way to more private ventures, he is once again out front promoting the economic importance of disability advocacy.

His has been a long and interesting road.

The formative years

Born in 1937 in New York City, Evan is the older of Evan and Francesca Moore Kemp's two children. His sister, also named Francesca, was born in 1940.

In 1941, Evan, Sr., moved his family to Cleveland, where he began what became his Saw and Knife specialty company, a manufacturing firm. The family and the business did well in those early years, and life was good. Slowly, however, Francesca Kemp began to notice the subtle physical struggles Evan had with balance and motion. His overall strength was deteriorating, and by the time he was ten he started to fall unpredictably. By 1945, an extensive medical inquiry had unfolded. Francesca needed to explore the reasons for this curious situation.

Although the family tried to promote a typical life experience for Evan, doctor visits and tests became the norm, not just in Cleveland, but beyond, to the more sophisticated cities of New York and Philadelphia. Francesca knew something was amiss and was determined to discover the root of the problem.

In spite of these physical struggles, however, Evan still managed to do well in school and was socially active. Although he was a good student, he struggled with certain topics, such as math and science. Years later, he would realize that these difficulties were due to dyslexia, but during his high school years he merely thought he needed to work a little harder to keep up.

As a young boy, Evan closely observed family and friends. Indeed, his keen sense of observation is a strength he claims serves him well in business today. One relative whom he observed and greatly respected was his uncle, David Meck, a judge in the Cleveland municipal courts. With countless dinner discussions revolving around issues before the court, Evan was convinced that law was for him. He would sit in Uncle David's courtroom, listening closely to the legal and judicial banter of the trials, and then later at family discussions, he would talk about the trials and legal tactics used by the attorneys he had observed.

Despite his increasing loss of strength, and those damn falls, Evan continued to participate in school and community activities. He played Little League baseball and held his own with his teammates. Nevertheless, his family continued to hunt for the cause of his problems.

Then, in 1949, when Evan was just twelve years old, after countless medical exams and assessments, Francesca and Evan Kemp, Sr. were finally given a diagnosis: their young son, Evan, they were told, had amyotrophic lateral sclerosis, the dreaded Lou Gehrig's disease. Worse, they said he would not live more than two additional years. They were devastated! How do you deal with news like that? What do you say or do? How do you cope with a death sentence for your own son?

These were bleak and deeply mournful days for the Kemp family, but they were not about to give up. Something had to be done. Maybe the Philadelphia physicians were wrong. Maybe a treatment could be found. Something could be done. Something must be done.

This situation, however, did not take the spirit out of Evan Kemp. Indeed, if anything, this "death sentence" of ALS strengthened his resolve to focus on goals and to make moments count. In fact, if there was any clarifying moment in his formative years that has influenced the man Evan Kemp is today, it was his refusal to give in to the struggle. As he came upon life's impasses, he often remembered this deep notion of only having two years to live. The dark shadow gave way to a focused and intense honesty about feelings and situations. The death sentence turned into a gift.

Francesca Kemp's relentless refusal to accept her son's death sentence led way to a stunning discovery, just two years later. After another round of tests, a Cleveland Clinic physician discovered that Evan did not have ALS at all. Rather, the family learned, he had a rare strain of muscular dystrophy.

The family's celebration, however, was tempered by their growing realization of muscular dystrophy. They learned that M.D., too, could lead to an early death for Evan. There was cause for hope, though. The muscular dystrophy that Evan had was not precisely diagnosed, and there might be the possibility of treatment or cure.

This reality rekindled Francesca Kemp's fighting spirit, and the entire family rallied to address the specter of muscular dystrophy. By 1946, they had initiated the Cleveland chapter of the Muscular Dystrophy Association (MDA). As they joined with others around the country, they helped create what is now the national Muscular Dystrophy Association. The family hosted countless dinners, held fundraisers, and began to vault the awareness of muscular dystrophy into the public consciousness. Perhaps if enough attention and research were given to this challenging disability, a treatment or cure that could benefit Evan might be found.

Indeed, an early boon to the MDA Movement was the Kemps' incorporation of the columnist and influential author, Drew Pearson of the *Washington Post*, who was Francesca's brother. He had a large public following with his columns and his books, *The Senator*, and *The Nine Old Men*, among others. His regular political column wielded deep influence over Washington, D.C. and the entire political framework of the country. He was controversial, outspoken and, in a way, feared by many a politician and bureaucrat for his propensity to flesh out the truth.

Once Drew Pearson was factored in, the visibility of muscular dystrophy and the Muscular Dystrophy Association took off. Through articles, and activities surrounding his nephew, Evan, Drew Pearson caused the nation to learn about muscular dystrophy, and disabilities in general. His presence and influence were critical to the initial success of the national Muscular Dystrophy Association's activities.

This close tie to Drew Pearson became another linchpin in the growth and ultimate career of Evan Kemp. Since the developing teenager had regular and steady contact with Uncle Drew, each man found himself influenced by the other. Drew Pearson learned more and more about muscular dystrophy and the character of his nephew. Evan, in turn, learned about the power and influence of newspapers and writings. He discovered that the pen is, indeed, mightier than the sword, a lesson that he still feels sets him apart from other disability advocates today.

As Evan progressed in his preparation for college, another interesting discovery unfolded. Although his grades were good, those challenging subjects of math and science continued to plague him. Finally the reason for his lifelong struggle with these subjects became clear. The answer came as more difficult news: he had dyslexia, as well as the muscular dystrophy label. Again, Evan tightened his focus and energy to deal with the dyslexia and prepare for college. He realized that he needed to train himself to think differently and deal with the dyslexia. With some tutoring support over the next few summers, he was able to maintain his grades, and by his junior year of high school, he scored 800 on his math SAT.

As he reflects on this experience today, Evan is convinced that training himself to think differently allowed other elements of his cognition to excel. He has always had an uncanny ability to remember things, and his wife, Janine Bertram, identifies his intellectual brilliance as a key element to his success. Evan considers his dyslexic condition a veiled gift that sets him apart.

These experiences of his youth combined to create a strong and unique character in young Evan Kemp. He learned the notions of advocacy and discovery from his mother and father. He found that if you work hard enough and continue to explore, a clearer path will unfold, that all dreams are possible with hard work. From his uncle, David Meck, he discovered a passion for law, justice and the rights of all people. This realization would set him on his life path as an advocate not only for people with disabilities, but also for others who are unjustly marginalized in society. From his uncle, Drew Pearson, he learned about influence and the actions for change that will rally people. He found that public expression in the press is always more powerful than public demonstration and disobedience. Finally, from his disabilities he discovered an inner strength and resolve. More than once during his life, he has found himself refocusing his position based on these lessons of life.

With all this in hand, Evan and his family began to explore colleges. They looked at a number of schools that would best prepare Evan for his future. His mother wanted him to stay close to home, but Evan was determined to have a typical college experience. Ultimately, they decided on Washington and Lee College in central Virginia, and on a warm August day in 1955, he set off to experience the next chapter in his life.

The learning years

The years 1955 to 1959 were exciting ones for America. Dwight Eisenhower was president and the United States was in the middle of an era of prosperity. Cities were booming, the suburbs were growing, and America was exploding with new products and ideas. Television reigned supreme and automobiles provided easy access to all parts of the country. The computer was invented on a campus in Illinois, and although we would not feel its intense impact for many years, the speculation about its application conjured up visions of a sci-fi tomorrow.

But all was not perfect. The Cold War with Russia, China, and other communist countries had escalated to a level where Americans were increasingly vigilant and fearful. America's young vice president, Richard Nixon, had his "kitchen debate" with the Russian premier, Nikita Khrushchev, and toward the end of 1958, fears abounded that the potential globalization of communism might become a real threat to democracy.

A U.S. Senator from Wisconsin, by the name of McCarthy, was creating havoc across the land with his attempts to flush out communists. McCarthy's favorite targets were film, television, radio and newspaper people who were thought to be sympathetic to the Communist party. As Senator McCarthy turned his attention from producer to director to actor, those people and groups connected to the media became frozen with fear. One such group was the Muscular Dystrophy Association.

Drew Pearson was, at this time, the chief spokesperson for MDA. Through his many columns and high visibility, he had acquainted America with muscular dystrophy. He also was more popular than ever as a columnist and an outspoken reporter. He was an easy target for McCarthy's anti-communist activities and the MDA was concerned that Drew Pearson and his controversial style, might lead the action to them. Such exposure would be disastrous to the Muscular Dystrophy Association and its fundraising capacity. Quietly at first, the MDA board of directors raised the issue; Pearson must go. Allies of Pearson could not believe it. Drew Pearson was as American as they came. Sure, he was outspoken and critical, but he had always stood strong for American ideals.

Still, the concerns of the MDA board persisted and deepened, as the sting of McCarthyism became more widespread. Then, without warning, the MDA leadership decided to drop Pearson from his role as MDA spokesperson. Overnight, it seemed, the dissociation occurred. This action stunned the Kemp family and outraged Evan, who was now attending Washington and Lee. The message was clear — controversy can be costly. The pain and anger generated by the MDA's unfairness to his Uncle Drew is still felt by Evan Kemp today.

Undergraduate school went well for Evan. He adjusted for his dyslexia with hard work and support from fellow students, and managed good grades in all his classes. He did, however, continue to struggle with falls and diminishing physical strength. A number of times, he talked to his physicians about using a wheelchair, but each time they advised against it. Their concerns seemed to relate more to the social consequences than the physical ones. Wheelchairs signified weakness and inability. Indeed, Franklin Delano Roosevelt, who used a wheelchair during his presidency, was never permitted to be photographed in his chair. His advisors were convinced that Americans would lose confidence in their leader if they viewed him in a wheelchair. So, Evan Kemp stuck to the grindstone and tried to remain open to the advice he was getting.

Even with his disability, Kemp was popular on the beautiful Washington and Lee campus. He had many friends and led a very active campus life. He attended the many cultural events and thoroughly enjoyed the stimulating banter the university offered. He had chosen Washington and Lee in a deliberate fashion. His family had encouraged him to consider schools closer to Cleveland or the Ivy League colleges in the northeast, but Kemp was drawn to the beautiful rolling hills of central Virginia. In addition, Washington and Lee had an excellent reputation for preparing students for law school, still a goal for young Evan Kemp. His desire to address social injustice was front and center in his plans.

As Kemp settled in at Washington and Lee, one key issue beginning to consume the American psyche was that of civil rights. Throughout the country, the fuse of discrimination and Jim Crow laws burned on. The Montgomery bus boycott, *Brown vs. Topeka Board of Education*, the Little Rock 9, and other civil rights activities, both formal and informal, began to capture the attention of Americans, and Evan Kemp was among them.

In fact, Evan had been well-primed to get on the civil rights bandwagon. As a young boy, his mother and father had exposed him to the dangers of discrimination. The elder Mr. Kemp spoke often about the race riots in Tulsa, Oklahoma where he had grown up, and how these riots split the community and drove a wedge between people. Mrs. Kemp constantly talked about the similarities we all share, rather than focusing on the differences. All people, she often reminded him, have a common bond regardless of their differences.

In a way, Evan felt a kinship with American blacks who were judged on their skin color. He knew the unfairness of this perspective from the way he was treated based on his muscle weakness and falling. He knew he had as much to offer as the next person, but he was still, at times, prejudged based on his physical situation. A passion for civil rights still burns deep in Evan Kemp, and he talks often about the civil rights approach to disability discrimination in his work today.

Kemp worked hard at Washington and Lee. He did not let his falling, which was becoming more frequent, get in the way of his college activities. Through his presence, Evan gained a solid respect among his university peers, and in 1958, his senior year, he ran for student body president. Although he did not win the seat, the taste for politics was established and Kemp furthered his understanding of the power of politics.

In 1959, Kemp received his Bachelor of Arts degree from Washington and Lee University, and although he was destined for law school, he felt the need to test himself and learn more about the world. And so, fresh out of school, he and his boyhood chum, David Robinson, headed off for Europe and the adventures that only two friends can find. David and Evan had been best friends since the early days in Cleveland. They played around in high school, and although David went off to Dartmouth when Evan headed to Washington and Lee, they still kept in close contact and shared similar thoughts.

Of course, they also had a plan. They hoped to capitalize on Evan's relationship to Drew Pearson, and Pearson's employment with Bell Syndi-

cate, a national wire service. They thought by researching the topic of social-
ized medicine and national health care, they could publish their findings
through Bell Syndicate. They were sure that the stories would be of interest
to Americans, and they could make some money as well. Unfortunately, they
were wrong. Although some initial stories were written, none were ever
published, and by 1960, after roaming most of Europe, the two friends found
themselves in Paris, flat broke.

Undaunted, they scoured the *U.S. Herald Tribune*, the American newspaper published daily in Europe, and found a want ad from an investment
firm looking for European representatives. David and Evan answered the
ad, and soon they were selling mutual funds in Europe and making a decent
wage. Their European adventure taught them valuable lessons about culture, language, customs, and style. It also taught Evan Kemp about the
world of investments, a lesson that would later serve him well in his career.
Perhaps even more importantly, Kemp found that as different as Europeans
were, their similarities to Americans, and all other cultures for that matter,
were telling. Europe had been a good experience, but by 1961, both men
were ready to come back home to begin to plan the rest of their lives. In
September of that same year, Evan Kemp enrolled in law school at the
University of Virginia.

Upon his return, he had thought about Harvard or Yale as law school
possibilities, but two things swayed him back to Virginia. One was the
beautiful countryside of Charlottesville. After four years at Washington and
Lee University, he just wasn't ready for the urban challenge of Boston or
New Haven. The second reason, however, was much more strategic. After
some research, he discovered that the University of Virginia undergraduate
and law schools had educated some twenty U.S. Senators. It was a perfect
launch pad for a person interested in politics and civil rights.

Law school at Virginia was filled with the excitement and passions of
the times. John F. Kennedy was in the White House and Camelot abounded.
We were still fighting communism, but the ugliness of the McCarthy era had
eased with the U.S. focusing its fears more narrowly in Southeast Asia. There
was a renewed sense of pride in being an American, and asking not what
our country could do for us, but what we could do for our country.

In this spirit, Evan Kemp consumed law school. He loved the challenges,
ideas and energies it brought. He also renewed acquaintance with an attractive woman named Ingrid Jonas. In fact, he first met Ingrid in Cleveland, at
a party given by his cousin Harriet, while on break from law school. They
immediately fell in love and became engaged. He was sure that once he
received his law degree, he would marry his fiancée, be immediately retained
by a large law firm, and find himself happily married in the throes of an
exciting legal career. He just couldn't wait. By his third year, however, reality
began to set in. In spite of his good grades, the large firms weren't interested
in him. Their honest appraisal was that a man with the weaknesses of
muscular dystrophy, who now had difficulty walking, would not have the
stamina or the public image they expected for big-time law. He should

consider something slower, more within the scope of a person with a disability. In interview after interview, some thirty-nine law firms gave him this same news. Discouraged by this reality, he decided to break off with Ingrid. He did not want to lead his fiancée down a path that was looking bleaker and bleaker. And so, with a University of Virginia law degree in hand, Evan Kemp picked up for Washington, D.C. He was hopeful Uncle Drew Pearson would be able to guide him into the next stage of his career.

The professional years

When Evan Kemp arrived in Washington, D.C. in October of 1964, the United States was deeply involved in the Vietnam war. President Lyndon Johnson was deploying more and more troops to Southeast Asia. Closer to home, the Beatles and the counter-culture had invaded the United States, and the turbulent '60s were in high gear. The Civil Rights Act of 1964 had just been signed and Dr. Martin Luther King was destined to win the Nobel peace prize.

Up until this point, Evan Kemp had been a Democrat. He supported the Kennedy/Johnson policies, was deeply devoted to civil rights, and held Dr. King up as a hero and mentor. People should be respected for the content of their character, not judged by the color of their skin or their physical status. He wanted to do his part in the movement for human rights, but first he needed a job. Enter again, Uncle Drew Pearson.

In spite of the brush with McCarthyism, Drew Pearson was a hugely popular American figure. His column, the *Washington Merry-Go-Round*, was syndicated in some 900 papers around the world. Additionally, he had a weekly broadcast on 225 ABC television stations every Sunday. Drew Pearson was well-respected.

As in the past, Drew Pearson was ready and willing to assist his nephew, and after a few calls, Pearson helped Evan land his first professional job, as an attorney with the Internal Revenue Service. It wasn't his dream job, but it was a start, and for three relatively unsatisfying years, he served as a tax law specialist with the IRS. Given his experiences in Europe, the position came easy to Kemp. He was well-versed in investment issues and found himself well in front of the IRS work demands. To fill in some of the increasing spare time he had, Evan became active in anti-war activities. In 1967, he was found in violation of the Hatch Act for recruiting signatures on an anti-war petition. As a federal employee, the Hatch Act prohibited political activities, but it didn't matter. The war was wrong and he needed to do his part.

He also began to connect socially in the Washington/Georgetown circles. He learned to play bridge, and through his aunt, Luvie Pearson, Evan met and made friends with new and influential people around Washington. Many of these new relationships would serve him well in the future.

On the personal side, Evan developed a key relationship with an attractive woman, Jane Copeland, who played in the bridge circles. Jane was bright and witty, and Evan found her intriguing. Within weeks of meeting, they became engaged. By September 1970, they were married, and Kemp couldn't have been happier. As a married couple, they made their way around the Washington social circles and time flew.

But the happiness was short-lived. In 1972, Jane developed a brain tumor, and after numerous exams, treatments, and surgery, their worst fears were confirmed — Jane's situation was hopeless, and the Kemps were told to expect the worst.

These were deeply trying times for Evan. He was in the midst of starting his career, but now was called to tend to his sick wife. By 1981, after more than eight years of care, it was clear that Jane would need a long-term-care facility. Evan searched long and hard, and finally chose a facility in North Carolina, which focused on terminal situations.

At the same time, Evan Kemp received some interesting news regarding his own disability. Since the age of fourteen, Evan and his family had believed his physical problems were related to muscular dystrophy. Further, because his physicians could not pinpoint the type of dystrophy, they had cautioned the Kemp family to expect the worse. His condition could continue to deteriorate and might lead to a premature death. Now, some sixteen years later, the truth had been discovered. After a battery of yet more tests, Kemp's physician found that Evan's symptoms met the profile of Engelburg Weylander Syndrome. This revelation was both liberating and frightening. Engelburg Weylander Syndrome is a rare neuromuscular disease similar to polio. Still, it could be progressive. Again, the uncertainty persisted.

By late 1967, Kemp learned about a law position open at the Securities and Exchange Commission (SEC). He jumped at the chance and won the job. Once with the SEC, he finally found the job satisfaction that had been lacking in other experiences. In his work, Evan became an expert in variable annuities and equities, and quickly rose through the ranks. He was respected among his peers and supervisors, and the future had never looked better. In 1972, however, while still at the SEC, an event occurred that literally changed Evan Kemp's life forever.

This story actually began with his requests to the SEC for simple accommodations for his continued struggle with muscle weakness and falling. As his Engelburg Weylander Syndrome condition evolved, Evan requested a parking spot in the SEC garage. He felt that being out of the elements and parking closer to the office would be safer and easier for him. His requests, however, had been denied. To get closer to the office, Evan found that if he parked near the garage and then walked through it, he could gain easier access to his office. The pattern seemed to work until that fateful day in 1971. On that June day, Evan arrived as usual. After locking his car, he proceeded down the parking ramp as he had always done, to short-cut through the garage. As he approached the doorway, he was not aware that the automatic garage door was beginning to close. Before he knew it, the door slammed down on him and violently threw him to the ground. By this point in his life, Evan Kemp was no stranger to falling. Since he was eight years old, falling had been a part of his life. This fall, however, was different. He was struck in the head and shoulder, and when he fell to the ground, his leg was wrenched under him, shattering it in the process.

Ending up in the hospital for three weeks with a broken leg, double vision, and a minor head injury, this would become the last fall Evan Kemp would experience. After twelve more weeks of rehabilitation, it was evident he would permanently need a wheelchair. The result was both symbolic and ironic. Finally, he would have the chair that would save him from the falls, but as a man and professional, he would forever be treated differently. He was now, truly, a disabled man.

Back at the SEC after the accident, everything had changed. Accolades for his performance that had been common before the accident, now stopped. Additionally, the management training opportunities he had sought all but ceased. Finally, when he bid for a new job that would enhance his career and develop his supervisory skills, he was flatly denied the opportunity. Evan could see no other explanation other than that the SEC felt a man with an obvious disability could not effectively supervise other people. This implication outraged Kemp, and he sought the counsel of those around him. It was Agnus Graham Meyer, a close friend of Drew Pearson and Allie Stevenson, who urged Evan to challenge the SEC. Agnus, who had struggled with a severe arthritic condition, had also been discriminated against by airlines which would not accommodate her special flight needs. Her perspective on this type of civil rights discrimination caused Evan to see this situation beyond the personal ramifications. It was symbolic of how society saw people with disabilities. In 1974, he filed suit against the SEC for discrimination.

He won the suit, but things at the commission would never be the same, and Evan knew he would need to shift professional gears. Indeed, Kemp's new disability reality began to introduce him to others in the "disability rights movement" who had to deal daily with the albatross of attitudinal barriers. It was clear to these advocates that it wasn't their disabling conditions that were limiting, but the perspectives of people around them. The "disability rights movement," as it had come to be known, was initiated in the early '60s. In various pockets around the country, courageous people with disabilities began to compare their situation to that of African-Americans in their quest for civil rights. As the civil rights pioneers began to move from the back of the bus, people with disabilities, languishing in nursing homes and other types of institutions, began to realize that they couldn't even get on a bus. As the Little Rock 9 pushed for integrated education, people with disabilities, and their advocates, realized they didn't have access to public education at all. Nowhere did the fires of inequity burn stronger about this discrimination than in Berkeley, California. Here, a young man named Ed Roberts lay in an iron lung, a prisoner of polio.

At the time, Ed Roberts was a student at the University of California by day and a nursing home resident by night. He was relegated to a world that treated him as a medical entity. Forget Jim Crow — Ed Roberts had no rights at all. Like most reformists, however, Ed had a strong and vivid mind. As he watched the nightly news parade of civil rights activities, he realized two important things. One was that civil rights is a concept that should apply to all people, including people with disabilities. More important, however, was that the road to civil rights is found in organization. With this realization, a movement was forged.

Ed Roberts lost no time in starting this movement. With colleagues at the University of California, he founded the first Disabled Student Services. This organizational energy soon spread, and shortly thereafter, the first Center for Independent Living (CIL) was founded in Berkeley. (It is important to note that in parallel, yet unrelated activities, the development of CILs, as they are known, was occurring in Boston and Champaign, Illinois.)

As with the other civil rights movement, the CILs' efforts in the late '60s were slow and tedious. Old norms change, and are adjusted to slowly, and are resisted every step of the way. Add the powerful and ingrained stigmas associated with people who have obvious, severe physical disabilities, and the concept of equality becomes that much more difficult. Consequently, the movement jelled slowly. Money was hard to come by, as government agencies did not trust people with disabilities. Their perspective was that people with disabilities were to be treated and helped, not funded directly. An even more fundamental problem was not having a name and identity from which to build.

Roberts and other national leaders with disabilities went around the horn on the issue of identity. A focused definition was needed to capture the movement's goal, but the format of the movement also needed to be separate from traditional rehabilitation efforts.

Kemp's frustration, like that of most of the others in the disability rights movement, was simple: here was a man who, prior to the accident, was a respected and active attorney; now, with the reality of a wheelchair, he was often treated as a nonentity. The stereotype and stigma held by others were enormous. Although he didn't feel different, the changed perspectives of those who met him were real.

These off-putting experiences were penetrating. Now that he was personally a subject of discrimination, he was reminded of experiences that had happened to others. Civil rights, women's rights, and religious rights were all situations that had new meaning. As he reflected more and more on his own experiences, it became clear that disability issues were human rights issues. As Kemp acclimated to the "disability arena," he found himself approached to join support or advocacy groups, or to band further with the cause. He was bright, articulate, vocal, and networked. He was a natural for the developing "disability rights movement." But he was never a real joiner, and even though he found acceptance with others who shared the cause, he mostly kept to his own path. Sure, he had played leadership roles in virtually every venue he had been in, but he was cautious about joining for joining's sake.

At this point in time, the disability movement was gaining ground. With the trailblazing work of Ed Roberts in California, and Fred Fay in Boston, more and more attention was being garnered for the independent living movement. Following the lead of civil rights, disability rights leaders such as Frank Bowe, Judy Heumann, Lex Frieden, David Williamson, Ed Roberts, Fred Fay, and others were defining "independent living," and pushing for legal rights for access, employment, and transportation. Frank Bowe's path-finding books, *Handicapping America* (1970) and *Rehabilitating America* (1975), laid the foundation for explaining and articulating the systematic and economic disempowerment of people with disabilities.

In Houston, Texas in 1974, major disability leaders came together to adopt a formal definition of the term "independent living," and set a course for advocacy that would amend the Rehabilitation Act of 1975. This amendment was groundbreaking because it was the first formal acknowledgment that disability issues were not of a medical nature, but a social one. Advocates had announced, loud and clear, that disability was a natural course of the human endeavor.

Certainly, the disability movement energized Evan Kemp. Along with the political and social realities that led to economic and social disempowerment, he also knew that part of the problem was the medical dominance of how people with disabilities were treated. Kemp found over and over, that the "sick role" prevailed in how he and other folks with disabilities were treated and served. He and his friends with disabilities often found themselves being considered sick, deficient, and defective. Kemp, however, along with many other advocates, did not see himself from either of these perspectives.

Still, the barriers, both attitudinal and architectural, were real for him. Along with being treated from a "sick role," he found that his wheelchair posed enormous barriers to places and things he had taken for granted prior to his accident. Simple steps, curbs, doorways, and other inaccessible settings clearly signaled he was not welcome at most places. These barriers were as loud as the previous generation's signs that said, "No colored allowed." He knew that this discrimination was a civil rights issue. From this point on, he became ardent about fighting the status quo. He was not sick, deficient, or abnormal, and he wouldn't give up his life for others' mistaken beliefs about people with disabilities.

In the late '70s, while still at the SEC, Kemp began to experience a sense of connectedness to certain players in the disability movement. Among them were Mary Jane Owens, Frank Bowe, and Deborah Kaplan. Indeed, it was Debbie Kaplan who introduced him to Ralph Hodgkins, the man responsible for advocating the use of airbags in cars. In turn, Ralph Hodgkins encouraged Evan to join the newly developed disability rights coalition founded and launched by his friend Ralph Nader. This invitation ushered in a whole new direction for Kemp, that of being a disability advocate.

The advocacy years

In 1980, America started its initial turn toward the political right with the election of Ronald Reagan as president of the United States. Reagan's fundamental platform was to begin the assault on government dominance and regulations. A new type of federalism was launched that initiated the use of block grants, and a focus on what was called "trickle-down economics." Using a free market focus, the Reagan Republicans argued that the private sector could do things better and more efficiently than government.

Indeed, in popular culture, there was an emerging conservatism that was equally influential. Defense and national patriotism were on the rise. The word "liberal" became a type of slur. Music and films began to shift to more fundamental themes. In Lynchburg, Virginia, Reverend Jerry Falwell began his "Moral Majority," a political action group with an emphasis on fundamental Christian values.

Some of these concepts appealed to Evan Kemp. He had grown increasingly conservative through the late '70s and felt that some of his more radical fellow advocates in the disability movement were on the wrong track. Certainly there were wrongs levied on people with disabilities, but the government quota/handout approach seemed too patronizing. Following some of the popular conservative logic that was sprouting up in race relations, Kemp began to align himself with the notion that government handouts and dependencies could be limiting and confining for people with disabilities. Although minorities needed to have individual opportunities for rights and justice, simply being a member of a particular group should not be the litmus test for handouts. In fact, it was the handouts that continued to perpetuate the cultural stigma of deficiency for people with disabilities.

In 1981, Kemp formally joined the Disability Rights Center (DRC). Founded by consumer advocate Ralph Nader, the DRC was interested in civil rights issues experienced by people with disabilities, and this offered a perfect fit for Evan Kemp, the advocate. Kemp liked Ralph Nader. He was principled, disciplined, and terribly egalitarian; all good things, and even though they differed on some points of view, Kemp reveled in his new job. In this role, Kemp found himself at the core of emerging debates, and nose-to-nose with key political and bureaucratic players. This offered an exciting change from the work at the SEC. Soon he was asked to direct the Center.

At the Disability Rights Center, Kemp did a myriad of things. He wrote testimony and opinions, constantly attended meetings, and represented disability issues at public and private gatherings. He met many new people.

One important introduction, a contact that would change his life and refocus his future, was with then-vice president, George Bush. The newly elected vice president was on the rise as a prominent and worldly politician. He had served in Congress, had been Director of the CIA, and had just emerged from an unsuccessful, yet engaging, run for the presidency. The two men met when Kemp, as DRC representative, joined the President's Commission on Deregulation, a commission chaired by George Bush. Kemp's job was to ensure that disability issues were represented.

Kemp immediately liked George Bush. He found a decency and sincerity that would ultimately endear the two men to each other. He also found many similar political perspectives. In spite of this alliance, however, Kemp felt that he was able to stay clear-headed and unbiased on disability issues while on the Commission. On a number of matters, he and Bush vehemently disagreed. Yet the friendship continued. One key area upon which they initially disagreed was Section 504 of the Rehabilitation Act. Bush wanted to make significant changes to this important legislation, but over time, Kemp convinced Bush not to dilute the protection this measure afforded people with disabilities. This victory and the Bush-Kemp alliance set the groundwork, some would argue, for the Americans with Disabilities Act (ADA), which Bush would sign some ten years later as the president of the United States.

As an advocate, Kemp felt that the one major area that separated him from his peers in the "disability movement" was his understanding of the media and the press. Being so close to Uncle Drew had taught him many lessons, but probably the most powerful was the understanding of how to get, and focus, press coverage, editorials, and opinion pieces on advocacy-related issues. Further, his assignments at the Disability Rights Center allowed him to hone his writing skills. Time and again, Evan has used the power of the pen to make a public point, but the most visible press experience happened in 1981.

One of Kemp's revelations, after he became a regular wheelchair user, was how much pity factored into disability issues. He began to feel it almost the day he started to use a chair. Over and over, he found that many people he met pitied him. Some were soft in their approach, and some were overt. Some people he met told him how courageous he was. Others treated him as if he were a child who was trying very hard to overcome his "handicap." This not only personally bothered him, but he also knew that if people are pitied, it is very difficult for them to also be respected — and rights are about respect, not pity.

By 1981, Kemp had had it with the pity approach, and decided to speak out. To him, the ultimate measure of pity for people with disabilities is found with telethons, and the king of the telethons was the Jerry Lewis Labor Day gathering for muscular dystrophy. So, using the power of the pen, Evan Kemp wrote a powerful editorial on telethons and planned to submit it to *Newsweek*. It was a 1300-word essay about pity, telethons, and how the image actually hurts people with disabilities as they attempt to involve themselves in the greater community. Kemp laid it all out. He wrote about how patronizing telethons are to people with disabilities; how the approach portrays folks with disabilities as poor, pathetic, and unfortunate. He stated that it was this national image that continued to keep people with disabilities devalued and stigmatized. He said that people with disabilities did not want to be "Jerry's kids."

As the Kemp article made its way into the *Newsweek* system, it caught the eye of a bright young editor from the *New York Times*. He quickly recognized the impact and potency of the piece, and called Kemp. He told him he liked the article and wanted to use it for the *New York Times* as an opinion piece, but it was too long. He asked Kemp to edit it, but he needed to have it in two hours in order to make the next day's *Times*. Kemp jumped at the chance and in less than two hours, the piece was in the editor's hands.

The editorial exploded into the general community. Kemp had touched a nerve and set off a national debate that still rages today. People all over the country began to respond. Human services agencies, media types, charitable foundations, and the general public joined in. Nowhere, however, was the explosion stronger than in the "disability community." Some were tremendously inspired. Evan Kemp had written what many had been feeling for years. Finally, someone had the courage to speak out. Others were outraged. How could a man, who had obviously benefited from the results of the MDA telethon, be so negative?

But the greatest rage was that of Jerry Lewis. Neither he nor the Muscular Dystrophy Association could believe how a person with a disability, and someone who was so closely aligned to MDA (Kemp's family had founded the chapter in Cleveland and were active on the early national MDA board), could say such things. Lewis responded publicly with strong actions. He personally and publicly accused Evan Kemp of being ungrateful. Comments followed about Kemp's selfishness and how his editorial had hurt other people with disabilities, most of whom were not as well off as Kemp.

Along with the public attacks, Kemp later discovered that shortly after his *New York Times* opinion piece, some people associated with the MDA had hired a private investigator to follow him to find ways to discredit him. The "investigator," a man named Steve Lockwood, initially established a friendship with Kemp, and then looked for ways to undermine his advocacy work on Capitol Hill and around the country. Kemp, who later had a chance to get to know Steve Lockwood outside of his "investigator" role, learned that Steve was paid close to $250,000 by MDA. When interviewed by *Vanity Fair* reporter Leslie Bennetts in September 1991, the "investigator," who only granted the interview on the grounds he not be identified, reported that MDA told him that the Kemp opinion piece had cost them over $4 million dollars annually in lost pledges. By discrediting him, they were determined to assure that Kemp did not do more damage. Indeed, the battle went on between Kemp and the MDA well into the early '90s. In his recent book, *King of Clowns*, Jerry Lewis devotes over ten pages to the Kemp controversy. His bitterness is clear. Immediately after the initial controversy over the editorial, Jerry Lewis did a temporary flip-flop. He and the MDA officials thought that by inviting Kemp to appear on the telethon, it might ameliorate the damage. Lewis met with Kemp prior to the telethon in Las Vegas to "feel" him out. As the two men talked over dinner, Lewis was tentative. He wanted Kemp to somehow soften his viewpoint, but knew he could not tell him what to say. When the telethon aired, Kemp appeared on camera in a short interview. He used the time to talk about the independent living movement and the advances of people with disabilities. He clearly kept his strong perspective of choice, control, and opportunity as cornerstones of the movement.

All went off without much of a hitch. Kemp kept his ground, and Lewis was not very happy. Some in the movement thought Evan had been too soft on the issue, that he should have used the time to blast further into the telethon controversy. Others felt that major information on the independent living movement was introduced to mainstream America. Most annoyed, however, was Kemp's mother, Francesca. Ever since the MDA dumped her brother, Drew Pearson, she had been bitter. After all the work she and her husband had done for the cause, the MDA officials not only maligned her brother, but barely said thanks. She refused to watch her son's interview on the telethon.

In late 1983, George Bush began to call on Evan Kemp for information and advice on disability issues. His first request was for Kemp to help him with a speech he had to make to a disability audience. Evan agreed, and the result was a powerful, sensitive talk for George Bush, and a satisfying writing experience for Evan Kemp. In fact, out of all the writing he has done in his career, Evan feels that this speech was one of his finest moments.

These requests and responses between Vice President Bush and DRC Director Evan Kemp set the tempo for a relationship that some might argue was the key element to Bush's ultimate success in the presidential election of 1988. (It was clear that the disability vote was a key constituency won by Bush in 1988. Given the close margin between George Bush and his opponent, Massachusetts Governor Michael Dukakis, some political analysts contend that without this constituency vote, Bush would have lost the election.)

In 1984, Ronald Reagan was re-elected by a large margin over rival Walter Mondale, and the conservative agenda was in full bloom. "Reaganomics" and new Federalism activities, such as block grants, were now a reality, and the call for deregulation continued to refine government. Evan Kemp was climbing the political and social ladder in Washington among the Reagan/Bush Republicans. With his clear articulation of disability minority issues that appealed more and more to the Republican strategists, as well as his regular bridge games with the likes of Boyden Gray and other key Republican advisors, Kemp was winning influential friends and making a real impact on key political leaders.

Indeed, the 1984 election between Reagan and Mondale was a key point of political clarification for Evan Kemp. As he considered the candidates, Kemp felt more and more a connection to the Reagan policies. The more he listened to the Democrats, the more he felt a paternalism that was degrading. It seemed that the Democratic candidates did not see folks with disabilities as peers, but as poor unfortunates who needed to be helped. This perspective began to grate into his core.

On November 12, 1984, Kemp made his way to the polling place in his northwest Washington, D.C. community. As he remembers it, the ten-minute trip took him an hour. He had been a lifetime Democrat from a strong, influential Democratic family. He had always voted Democratic. And yet this day, as he made the slow, deliberate trip to the polls, Kemp finally decided to vote for Ronald Reagan for president of the United States.

Two weeks later, Kemp changed his party affiliation from Democrat to Independent. By early 1985, Evan Kemp was a registered Republican. As his political views became more conservative, at least on minority issues, it was clear that Evan would need to reconsider his role at the Disability Rights Center. He found that more and more of the expectations followed a route with which he did not agree. He left his position shortly after the Reagan victory, and reviewed his options. After thorough exploration, Evan decided to teach law on a part-time basis at Catholic University in Washington, D.C. and to assess other options as they became available. He found going back to law school, albeit from a teaching point of view, to be as invigorating as his student experience.

His tenure as a law professor was short-lived, however. In 1987, President Reagan nominated Evan Kemp for a seat on the Equal Employment Opportunities Commission (EEOC), which was chaired by Clarence Thomas. This appointment was an opportunity he could just not pass up. It offered a chance to serve his president, continue contact with George Bush, and to get closer to Clarence Thomas, an influential African-American whose views he respected.

Although Evan Kemp was well known and well respected in political circles, his confirmation was not the smooth sailing he had expected. The major opponent to his nomination was Senator Howard Metzenbaum of Ohio. As a strong liberal, Metzenbaum was concerned with Kemp's growing conservative notions. Indeed, most disability advocates seemed to be liberal by nature, and the liberal political leaders, like Metzenbaum, were wary. To address these concerns Evan decided to be proactive rather than reactive. Knowing of Metzenbaum's interest and connection to blindness and visual issues in his home state of Ohio, Kemp called some of his blind friends. He explained his posture to these advocates and persuaded them to support his nomination. They in turn contacted Senator Metzenbaum, and soon he changed his posture on Evan Kemp. Within a week, Kemp won Senate confirmation to the EEOC.

Once confirmed and in his new role, Kemp navigated well through conservative Washington, D.C. He felt strongly about the issue of civil rights, but aspects of affirmative action and quotas did not seem effective or appropriate. Serving on the EEOC helped sharpen and focus his views on civil rights and equality. Evan learned much from his experiences with the EEOC. As he attended meetings and forums, he honed skills, articulated arguments, and found more and more viability from the emerging Republican approach to cultural injustice. Central to the theme was economic empowerment. Kemp was convinced that the more folks with disabilities had opportunities to develop businesses and access jobs, the sooner equality would emerge. This same perspective was being argued for other minority struggles. The growing thesis was that the giveaway programs promoted by many Democratic leaders just perpetuated a dependency image, and further devalued minorities.

By the mid-1980s exciting things were happening in Evan Kemp's life. He was heavily sought after to speak and write, and was constantly on the go. He was meeting interesting people and reveled in the intellectual repartee. Then, on June 27, 1985, Kemp had another meeting that would again redirect his life.

It was that day in June when Kemp's good friend, Bob Funk, called on him for a favor. Funk and Kemp had become close in the Nader Disability Rights Center days, and though differing in political directions, they kept in regular contact. It seemed that Funk had two friends from Berkeley who were coming to Washington, D.C. to lobby for prison reform, and they needed a place to stay. He knew Evan had room and was always interested in meeting interesting people. And these were interesting people.

Janine Bertram, one of the visitors, was, and is, a story unto herself. Born and raised on the West Coast, Janine was caught up in the early swirl of the '60s protest era. First there was Vietnam, then the women's movement, and then a full, radical realization of the inequities of world. Protests led to more and more leftist concerns, and then ultimately to anarchist activities. By 1973, Janine was a member of the George Jackson Brigade, an anarchist group which took the name of George Jackson in symbolic defiance.

George Jackson was a petty criminal who was treated wrongly by what Bertram's group felt was a racist judicial system. The George Jackson Brigade was convinced that the only way to address the ills of society was to strike back. Somewhat aligned with the Symbionese Liberation Army, the George Jackson Brigade began to conduct acts of terrorism: first robberies, and then bombings. As the terrorist acts increased, the Jackson Brigade members found themselves needing to work from the political underground. Moving from place to place, Janine and her associates were always one step ahead of the law.

Then, while in Tacoma in 1978, Janine and a fellow brigade member made a stop at a local fast-food restaurant. Little did they know that a stakeout for them was getting closer and closer. At the restaurant, they were arrested and taken into custody. The long road underground was finally over. Bertram pled guilty and was convicted of bombing and bank robbery. She was given a ten-year sentence, and remanded to Pleasanton, California's correctional facility for women. There she served four and a half years behind bars. On her first day at Pleasanton, while in the cafeteria line, Janine found herself face to face with a fellow inmate serving soup — Patty Hearst, who was doing her own "hard time" for terrorist activities.

During this time, Janine became very interested in a program designed to support prisoners who were also parents. She was amazed at the difficulties and distinctions experienced by female inmates when it came to simple issues related to their children. It was commonplace for mothers to be denied basic parenting requests that were vital to their children's best interests. This project initiated a passion that still burns within Bertram.

By 1982, Janine had moved from Pleasanton to a halfway house. There she continued her prison reform work and began the long road back to mainstream community activities. In 1984, she moved to Oakland, California to work in a "prison match" program. The advocacy continued, and then on June 27, 1985, Janine found herself in the home of Evan Kemp, a friend of a friend. How interestingly fate moves.

Evan and Janine had an immediate connection. The first night they met, conversation continued until the wee hours of the morning. The days in Washington flew, and soon Janine went back to the Bay area to continue her work. But the bond had been forged.

Janine and Evan wrote letters at first and then began to phone. By July 26, Evan found himself on a jet to California. The relationship grew around their respect for mutual experiences, interest in their differences, and a strong desire to know more about each other. The visit ended far too soon, but Kemp was sure that he was falling in love. Back in D.C. in the fall, Evan and Janine wrote and called, and by January 10, 1986, Janine moved in with Evan at his Washington apartment, where they had first met.

Although he was an incredibly strong man, Janine Bertram totally re-energized Evan Kemp. They became caught up in each other's issues, as well as remaining focused on their private matters. They relished the constant flow of intellectual discussion and banter in the networks they had on their own, as well as the ones they were developing together. They agreed and disagreed on a myriad of issues, and they continue to display a healthy exchange of ideas. Although their passions seem different, in an odd way they are linked. Both have experienced the throes of devaluation and stigma. Both have had situations where institutions were dominant in their lives. Both have felt the joys of rebirth when given a chance to move out of the ugly light of stigma. Indeed, they have joked that they ought to collaborate on a book that they teasingly say should be entitled, *The Convict and the Cripple*.

By 1987, George Bush was deep into the process of being a candidate for president of the United States. More and more, he relied on Evan Kemp to help him mobilize a strategy to court the disability vote. Evan shared ideas, names, and focus, and George Bush listened. On January 21, 1989, George Herbert Walker Bush was inaugurated as the forty-fourth president of the United States. It was a close race with Governor Michael Dukakis, and some analysts, including the Harris pollsters, suggested that the margin of difference in the election was the mobilization of the disability vote.

After the election, Kemp was in the driver's seat. Doors were opened to him and he was ready for a greater challenge. Kemp was interested in the position of assistant attorney general in charge of civil rights. He made his interest known to Brad Reynolds, but discovered that Attorney General Dick Thornburgh had different thoughts. Kemp now understands that Thornburgh was concerned about appointing an activist to a key federal position. While President Bush was on a goodwill mission to China, Attorney General Thornburgh announced another candidate for the position of assistant attorney general.

At the same time, however, Clarence Thomas, chair of the EEOC, was also looking for a change. One of President Bush's first actions was to name Clarence Thomas to the D.C. Court of Appeals. This move was good for Thomas, but shot a hole in the EEOC. The Bush team approached Evan Kemp for the chairmanship. This role opened a whole new series of doors for him.

The EEOC had historically been an agency with problems. Over the years, it had gotten behind in cases, and in some circles it was considered to be inept and insensitive. That was before Clarence Thomas was named EEOC chair. In spite of the huge publicity Thomas received during his Supreme Court nomination in 1991, when Thomas inherited the EEOC, he literally transformed it. According to Kemp, under Thomas' stewardship, the EEOC began to reinvent itself. Database changes, adjustments to process, and policy updates were all made under his watch. When Kemp stepped in as the new chair, Thomas made a personal commitment to the transition. He met with Kemp on a regular basis to ensure that the EEOC revival would continue. Although Kemp had worked with Thomas before, his respect and friendship grew steadily at this time. Kemp continued the advances at EEOC until his resignation in April of 1993.

In 1990, with the successes around the world, and especially in the Desert Storm military campaign in the Middle East, it appeared that George Bush would be easily re-elected. He had a 92% approval rating and was well respected around the world. For Evan, this re-election would set the tone for so many changes he wanted to effect at the EEOC. They had deregulated many cumbersome policies, and Kemp was incredibly optimistic. Along with his work at the EEOC, he continued to lobby for economic opportunities for people with disabilities, and he was convinced of his direction.

Perhaps the most focused contribution Kemp feels he had made at this point was his role in promoting the ADA (Americans with Disabilities Act). Since his work at the Disability Rights Center, Kemp and other high-profile advocates knew a focused law was needed to enhance the civil rights of people with disabilities. Indeed, advocates had been working since the early 1960s to include disability issues into the general civil rights laws, but had met with opposition. At that time, many African-Americans felt that including disability issues into the general civil rights legislation would dilute the gains already obtained. And so, it became clear that something unique would have to be fashioned.

First came the Rehabilitation Act Amendments of 1973, and then 1978. These landmark changes addressed discrimination and established some due process. By the mid-1980s, a full-blown effort was underway to sculpt a separate law that could stand on its own and clearly announce to American society that folks with disabilities were an important segment of our country.

Early 1988 saw the introduction of the Americans with Disabilities Act into Congress. It was a bipartisan effort and immediately attracted attention. Supporters and opponents began to plan their arguments and the challenge began. As the majority of disability advocates tended to fall on the liberal side of the scale, Evan Kemp and Justin Dart, as Republican advisors on disability matters to George Bush, became important players in the process. Justin Dart was chair of the President's Committee on Employment of People with Disabilities. He had deep Republican roots and was well respected in the disability community.

Even if the ADA was passed by the Congress, it would have to be signed by the president, and it was looking more and more as if George Bush would be the next president. Kemp began to speak out on the need for ADA, but his perspective was keeping key features in the bill that would attract conservative support. This posture outraged the mainstream disability advocates. In fact, after a speech delivered at the President's Committee on Employment of People with Disabilities conference, Kemp was approached by five well-known disability advocates, who urged him to change his perspective. But Kemp had always been a man of conviction, and was convinced that the adjustments he advocated were not only essential for passage, but would create a better ADA.

By 1989, the adjusted ADA bill was well on its way to passage. It had passed the Senate, looked good in the House of Representatives, and had key administrative support. Although he was a top-level political appointee, Kemp continued his activism. He called other leaders, wrote opinions, and was clearly in charge of a movement to pass the ADA. Indeed, it was a great day in July 1990, when, in the White House Rose Garden, before some 5000 friends and fellow advocates, Evan Kemp introduced President George Bush, as he officially signed the ADA.

In 1992, in a close national election, George Bush lost the presidency to Bill Clinton, the governor of Arkansas. This election jolted Washington, and clearly set the tone for change, but it did not surprise Evan Kemp. Although he had maintained his friendship with the president during the campaign period, he was utilized less and less as an advisor. Unlike 1988, he had little input into the 1992 campaign, and as he sat at the Republican National Convention that year in Houston, he predicted that Bush would lose to Clinton.

This premonition was based on Kemp's keen political savvy. Two important things had swayed him. One was that George Bush had become increasingly preoccupied with foreign policy issues. His Gulf War popularity had convinced his key aides that domestic and civil issues were not as important as world politics. Consequently, Bush seemed to lose interest in keeping domestic issues, such as disability rights, as critical. After all, he was the president who had signed the ADA.

Kemp's other political hunch related to Bush's rival, Governor Bill Clinton of Arkansas. Kemp was no fan of Clinton, but was impressed and amazed when Bill Clinton took on, and beat, all political comers in Arkansas in the 1980s, most specific was his dominance over Kemp's friend, Jim Guy Tucker. Kemp and Tucker had met in the late 1960s, and although Kemp is not easily swayed, he was taken aback by Tucker's political savvy. He was impressed with Tucker's intelligence, style, and sensitivity. Kemp knew that Tucker would go far in politics, perhaps even as far as the presidency. Little did he realize then that Tucker's major political rival in his home state would be a young politician named Bill Clinton. Over and over again, Tucker and Clinton squared off for political positions and Clinton always won. Who was this man who could compete with Jim Guy Tucker and win? Now, this same man was running against his boss, and Kemp knew he would be a formidable candidate.

After the election change, a whole new cast of players descended on the Washington, D.C. scene, and Evan Kemp knew that his days at EEOC were numbered. Well known and well respected, Evan considered his options. He could teach law, or continue his work in advocacy. He could practice law or consider going into investment annuities, one of his many skill specialties.

Strangely, for a man who had spent the better part of his adult work life in the public sector, leaving government service was liberating to Kemp. He felt fortunate to have had interesting experiences but was now ready to move forward into the private sector.

After much review, Evan decided to go into private business. He set up some business programs and then with his friends, Bob Funk and Ann Colgrove, set up EKA Associates. Starting as a small medical supply operator, EKA is today a $12 million business with multiple services and offices. They are currently the largest dealer on the east coast with plans for further national and international expansion.

After a lifetime of success in government and business, Kemp reflected on the disability movement. There was still so much more to do, but he was optimistic about the future, especially when considering the young, new advocates who stand ready to take up the cause. With key victories in place, such as ADA, he looks forward to the things that remain to be done.

One issue is the hotly debated FDR Memorial for Washington, D.C. Kemp strongly favored that the memorial portray President Roosevelt in his wheelchair. Such an action would be symbolic of the abilities and contributions of folks who have disabilities.

Another important issue is physician-assisted suicide. As the debate for personal choice in society continues to develop, some people see choice applying to death, especially in situations where there is not much hope for survival. Kemp, however, has problems with this issue. He fears that some people might decide, for some people with disabilities, that death would be better for them. Indeed, in a recent situation in Saskatchewan, Canada, the Lattimer case, a father essentially took the life of his daughter, a thirteen-year-old girl with cerebral palsy, because he felt her life would just be too hard. After being arrested for murder, and twice convicted by a Canadian court, the majority of Canadians, in a public opinion poll, found him innocent and having done the "right" thing. Kemp, and many other disability advocates, found this to be incredibly unconscionable. The last issue, and one that Kemp has championed as his personal quest, is economic empowerment. For people to be truly valued, they must have access to viable economic power. Kemp advocates for business opportunities and chances for people who have been locked out of economic ventures. These, he believed, were the clear route to equality.

Before closing our series of interviews, I asked Evan Kemp to summarize what he saw as the key elements of leadership, not just in the disability arena, but in life. He paused, and looked out into his courtyard on this sunny spring day. The sun shone on him like wisdom. "First," he said, "you have to deeply believe in your cause. You must be strongly committed." Next, he said, "You must take time to hear the other person's point of view." Lastly, he cautioned, "Don't make unnecessary enemies. You never know when they might become your allies." Wise advice, indeed.

On June 22, 1996, Evan and his long-time companion, Janine Bertram, were wed in a simple church ceremony in Washington, D.C. Present were a few friends, including some homeless folks who spend time near the church. Janine is still active in her work with prison reform, while Evan remains focused on his business interests. These two very different people have bonded together in the spirit of wanting to change this country for the better. Although Janine still works the classic advocacy strategies, Evan is convinced that the route to full inclusion will be an economic one.

As Evan and Janine enter the next chapter of their individual and joint lives together, we paused one afternoon to reflect on their relationship and how Janine sees this man, Evan Kemp. I asked them how they are similar; one a former radical anarchist, the other a blue-blood economic entrepreneur. They looked at each other and then readily identified the following items:

- The drive to include excluded people.
- The importance of empowerment and personal value.
- A yearning for peace and brotherhood.
- An intolerance for capital punishment.
- An independence in political thought.

Then I asked the obvious follow-up, "On what issues do you differ?" They again paused, these two thoughtful and intellectual people, and then responded:

- Kemp has problems with paternalism.
- Bertram wants to build on what they have, rather than fix problems.
- Kemp is economically conservative.
- Bertram tends to be politically liberal.

As we continued our dialogue, I asked Evan Kemp to reflect on the "disability rights movement," one that he helped create and develop. Was he optimistic? Did he have any major concerns? Again he paused, looked out toward his garden, and told me that he is hopeful about the younger, emerging leaders in the field. It seems that some old fears have been overcome and that there are fresh dreams for the future. He cautioned, however, that attitudes still loom as the biggest challenge and barrier to equality.

Next, I asked him to summon up his proudest moment, and without hesitation, he said the ADA. He is glad to have been in a position to influence the president and to help shape this landmark law. He was quick to add, however, that gaining the ADA was not a one-person show. It took many dedicated years and a myriad of players. Still, it is a mark he helped make.

After the many trials and tribulations of his life, I asked Evan to reflect on leadership. Clearly he is a leader, and has spent his career around leaders. What did he feel were the hallmarks of leadership? Kemp offered three thoughts:

- A leader must have a belief and a deep personal commitment to that belief. Often the most challenging obstacle to change is when the leader holds on to his values in spite of opposition and resistance.
- A leader must work to see others' points of view. They might not adjust, adopt, or change, but they must seek to explore where other people are coming from.
- A leader must not make excuses when things don't take the shape that one wants.

As I prepared to leave that day, my final questions moved to the future. On the professional side, Evan felt that the notion of "economic integration" was the critical next step for people with disabilities. He was looking forward to continued work in this area, directly with EKA, and indirectly as an advocate in writings and speeches. He is convinced that the route to equality lies as much in the board rooms as it does in the court rooms.

On the personal side, he and Janine were excited about the summer and the continued dovetailing of their passions and dreams.

And so it goes. This man, Evan Kemp, who was expected to die as a teenager, who was challenged by a rare disabling condition that was not diagnosed until his adult years, who faced wanton discrimination throughout his entire life, found that life is deeply satisfying. He has made a rare contribution to his country and his culture — perhaps around the world. Through his writings, speeches, and tireless efforts, he has contributed ideas that will help create better lives for the many who will follow.

An amazing life, an amazing man.

It's curious, the bends and turns in life. Each day all of us are subjected to gifts that sneak up on us, as well as to the unexpected tragedies that occur. Most of the time they defy logic, always they take us aback. Such a turn happened to me as I was putting the finishing touches on this chapter. I was close to a draft that I planned to share with Evan and Janine, and had taken my notes and manuscripts with me as my family looked forward to spending a long weekend at the Delaware shore. As we rushed from the house early that August morning, I tossed my newspaper into the back seat, to read later at the shore. Our trip was smooth, and as my wife and I sat on our beach chairs later that day, I finally got a chance to read my paper. The sounds of laughter and surf and gulls were starkly muted as I saw the obituary of Evan

Kemp. Here in print was the review of the life of the man whom I had come to know, respect, and admire. The man I was joking with, just a few weeks before, as we became better acquainted. Now he was gone.

The high points of his career jumped out at me as I read the obituary, and in the silence of my mind, I could hear him saying the words, yet now he was gone. My thoughts moved to the sixtieth birthday party Janine had held for him just three months before, that had hailed "Come join us for a Not-Dead-Yet party for Evan."

As I sat on that beach and reflected on the life and times of Evan Kemp, my sorrow started to soften. Here was a man who lived in the shadows of death his whole life — who did more in his sixty years than most of us dream to be possible — who left a true set of tracks for future generations to follow. Here was a man who fought the odds, and won more than he lost — who carried his own burdens, yet kept his eyes on the prizes of equality and respect for all people. Here was a man who stood up for what he believed, even when powerful obstacles presented themselves.

I remembered that in our final interview, Evan had told me that he had no regrets about the turns of his life. He said that if he died tomorrow, he would go to his reward feeling that he had accomplished more than he had ever expected. And so it was to be.

I know that writers, especially biographers, must not get too close to the subjects of their work. Now, I don't consider myself to be a biographer, but I was called on to write this chapter and charged with being objective in getting a clear story. I started my work on this chapter in this spirit, and I believe I now close this effort with this same objectivity. But I must tell you that I came to like Evan Kemp. He was blunt, gutsy, and honest. In spite of his many accomplishments, he was never a braggart or a know-it-all. Brief as it was, I will miss this man and I feel better for our acquaintanceship.

And so it is, the life and times of Evan Kemp come to a close. He won't see this final draft, but I feel that if he had, he would have been pleased. Certainly he would have had some corrections; such is the bent of lifetime advocates. They believe that things can always be better. Still, I think he would look up from the document and say "not bad."

chapter three

Justin Dart, Jr.

Christine Reid

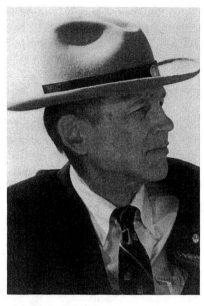

"Don't put in there that I'm the father or godfather of the ADA — it doesn't have one father or mother. It has hundreds!" Justin Dart, Jr., is a passionate leader of the disability rights movement. His contributions have been recognized through a multitude of honors and awards, including the highest civilian award in the United States, the Medal of Freedom, presented to him by President Clinton in 1998. Accompanying that medal was the following formal citation:

> "The purpose of human society," Justin Dart has said, "is to empower every individual to live life to his or her God-given potential." He has made that purpose his own. Since contracting polio as a young man, he has worked for the independence, inclusion and empowerment of people with disabilities. A leading architect of the Americans with Disabilities Act and a driving force behind its passage, he has had a profound impact on the public policy of this Nation. Justin Dart

> has earned our thanks for helping us recognize the
> possibility within each individual for tenaciously ad-
> vocating equal access to the American Dream for all
> our people.

Mr. Dart has said that this medal really recognizes the disability rights movement as a whole, not just himself as an individual. He explained, "I know that I am simply a symbol of those thousands of patriots who have fought and sacrificed for our cause over the years. Colleagues, this is your medal. I am the luckiest man in the world to have the privilege of working with you in the cause of justice…"

"I'm no saint."   Most people who knew Justin Dart, Jr., when he was a child would never have expected him to become a beloved and respected leader of anything. Dart has often said, "I was an obnoxious kid." He explained, "In a wealthy family, characterized by vicious competition among super-visible winners, I found identity as a super-visible loser."

Dart described his grandfather, Charles S. Walgreen, as initially "a pool shark, a kind of con man" as a young man. But, Dart said, at some point, Walgreen "became more ambitious," borrowing $500 to start a drugstore "based on treating people right — 'You're always welcome at Walgreen's.' It grew to be the largest drug chain in the nation." Charles Walgreen's wife, Myrtle, has been described by Dart as "my beautiful grandmother, a great lady who never forgot the simple principles of humanity and justice, even when she became very rich, very fast. She always had time to counsel me, to be with me in a way other people would not." Charles and Myrtle Walgreen's daughter, Ruth, became Justin Dart, Jr.'s mother.

Dart has written that his mother was a "brilliant…flaming liberal feminist writer" from the 1930s through the 1950s. "She published an avant-garde magazine and drilled into me the values of human rights when it was totally unfashionable. I remember the day when she said, 'Justin, it is *not* all relative. There *is* evil. We must fight evil." Ruth Walgreen married Justin Dart, Sr., who was considered by his son Justin, Jr., "quite different from my mother: a politically conservative businessman, a consistent Republican, an advisor to several Republican presidential candidates and presidents…" Ruth and Justin, Sr. had two children: Peter Dart, and Justin, Jr., who was born in Chicago in 1930.

Young Justin, Jr.'s first word was "football." His father had been an All-American football player, and competition was an important feature of the household. Justin, Jr. later described his family as a group of "passionate overachievers." He explained that not only was it unacceptable to be number two in anything, but even number one wasn't quite good enough "if you don't break a world record." Ruth and Justin, Sr. divorced in 1939.

When Justin Dart, Jr. was fourteen, he broke the all-time demerit record (previously held by Humphrey Bogart) at Andover, America's most famous preparatory school. He boasted, "I never met a person I couldn't insult. I never met a rule I couldn't break." Yet, he knew that "people didn't like me. I didn't like myself."

Dart contracted polio when he was eighteen. He was aware that "the doctors told my parents I was going to die in a few days, but not to worry, — I would be better off dead." His parents disagreed, and placed Justin, Jr. in a hospital "operated by Christian people to whom each life was sacred — people who were passionately dedicated to expressing love" for young Dart, who was moved by what he saw. "This was new for me. These people seemed so happy. I thought, Justin, if you are only going to live a few more days, why not try this love thing — try smiling and being positive. It worked."

"I count the good days in my life from the time I got polio." Dart explained that the loving attitude of those hospital workers "not only saved my life, they made it worth saving." While still in the hospital, Dart married his high school sweetheart, Suzanne Sloan, "a fine young woman who contributed much to my life — including three beautiful daughters" (Ruth Suzanne, Ann Linda, and Elizabeth Myrtle). Dart had experienced some healing of both body and spirit while in the hospital. Yet, when he came out of that institution at the age of twenty, he faced a society where there was "apparently no place" for a wheelchair user. He said, "I felt the power of love, but I didn't have the slightest idea how to use it…I was desperate for a formula to live."

Dart read a book by Mohandas Gandhi, *My Experiments with Truth*. From this work, he learned that "anybody can live well" and "reach greatness" without a lot of money, a title, or anyone else's approval. Dart explained, "The way you do that is to examine your own truth — what is it that you really believe — and then live it." He found that Gandhi's truth was "in advocating for a united, loving society, with justice for all." Dart said, "The simplicity, the power, the self-evident validity of this concept overwhelmed me," but also "gave me a vision, a passionate vision that permeated my whole consciousness and still does." Finding one's own personal truth and living it is "a pretty simple idea, but a profoundly powerful one; it mandates a lifetime of dedicated experimentation."

In 1951, Dart enrolled at the University of Houston as an education major. He had been advised that the University of Illinois would be a more accessible educational institution for a wheelchair user, but Dart was determined to go to a university where he would be "totally independent and not part of a program for people with disabilities." He explained, "I didn't want to be part of a program with a lot of rules and regimentation." To get to his classrooms in Houston every day, Dart sat in his chair at the bottom of each building's steps, asking fellow students or others passing by to carry him up the stairs. Distancing himself from his family and their money, Dart sought part-time employment while in college. Rejected throughout the city by other potential employers, Dart sold and delivered *The Houston Chronicle* daily newspaper, for two-cents gross profit each. Showing an entrepreneurial spirit, he increased sales on his delivery route by more than 40%.

In 1952, Dart founded the first organization to promote racial integration of the segregated University of Houston. He worked with leaders of the CIO, AFL, NAACP, and other liberal groups to form the Harris County (Houston) Democrats in 1953, authoring the group's constitution, organization plan, and precinct-organizing manual. The Harris County Democrats eventually took control of the party structure from the traditional, anti-civil-rights "Dixiecrats," and elected several members of Congress. During this time, however, Dart did not recognize the oppression of people with disabilities as a civil rights issue. He has said, "It is a dramatic example of the power of stereotype that I could be a passionate advocate for racial equality, and not be conscious of the discrimination that I was experiencing."

Dart was an honors student throughout his degree program, but during his senior year, he was informed that he would not be able to complete the requirements for a teaching degree because it was "not possible" for him to complete his supervised teaching practicum while using a wheelchair. Dart changed his major to history and education, and added to it a master's degree in history (completed in 1954). Ironically, as a graduate student, he taught several sections of required history and government courses for the University of Houston, from his wheelchair.

Dart started law school at the University of Texas in Austin in 1954 and was a member of the honor fraternity. After one and a half years in that program, he was "mostly just tired of studying," and anxious to go into business. He intended to pursue a career in business anyway, and had planned to get a law degree "to be my own lawyer for the business." But after he met a business lawyer who had never lost a case, he reasoned that it made more sense for him to employ a top lawyer and focus his own efforts on business instead of law. In retrospect, he recently said with a smile, "I should have finished. Many of my colleagues and opponents are attorneys, and get paid well."

"When I couldn't get a job, I started my own business."   When Dart looked for opportunities to launch his career in the business world, he found nobody willing to hire a wheelchair user. Even his family's company refused to hire him, saying there was "no room for the wheelchair behind drug store counters." So, Dart borrowed $35,000 to start his own bowling business in Austin. His facility featured the new automatic bowling (pin-setting) machines that revolutionized the business. The business became a prominent success, "#1 in the field in Austin." Dart worked hard, eighteen hours per day, sticking with the business even after he realized that too many competitors were coming into the area. He explained, "...taxes hit profits before repayment of the borrowed capital...," so it was difficult to get ahead, even with a successful enterprise. As soon as it was feasible, he sold the Austin business for a small profit, and "got in on the ground floor in Mexico," opening the first automatic bowling alley in Latin America. He was given a commendation by the president of Mexico for his role as the principal promoter of the Mexican national men's and women's bowling teams, which

were world champions in 1960. His Mexican bowling business was a great success, but "then really big competitors came in." Dart sold the business in Mexico while it was still profitable. For all his hard work in the bowling ventures, Dart ended up with a financial profit, but also a bleeding ulcer and a divorce from his wife, Suzanne. Since then, Dart has explained that Suzanne, "was extremely patient with all my wild activities, but we got divorced in 1962. That wasn't her fault — she married a pretty wild young man with a lot of problems — and she empowered me at a time when I had no other support."

"Plastic pots..."   At the same time Dart was looking for his next business venture, his father was looking for somebody to take Tupperware into Japan. Dart explained, "Nobody else wanted to do it." Tupperware had no patents in Japan, there were bureaucratic barriers for an American firm trying to run a business in Japan, and the manufacturing systems used to make the Tupperware products were expensive. After all, noted Dart, "They're guaranteed for life."

Justin Dart, Jr., took on this challenge, starting Japan Tupperware in 1963, with a total of four employees (including himself). The company grew in a couple of years to include more than 25,000 employees. Japan Tupperware was recognized by the Japanese Marketing Federation as an outstanding example of domestic marketing in Japan. Dart hired and promoted women as salespeople and managers in his corporation, an unusual practice in Japan at that time. Noticing the media attention given to the Paralympics in Tokyo in 1964, he launched a "help-the-handicapped" campaign, giving away wheelchairs and hiring a small group of young men with paraplegia who had previously been institutionalized. In addition to giving them opportunities to work in his factory, Dart taught the young men how to play competitive wheelchair basketball. Using wheelchairs, these young athletes won exhibition games against famous non-disabled teams. When they were scheduled to play against the non-disabled Japanese Olympic basketball team on national television, a public relations expert suggested to Dart and the Tupperware team, "Maybe you'd better take it easy. You might lose sympathy." Dart responded, "That's exactly what we want to do! Go to it, boys." The Tupperware team defeated the Olympic team, with a score of 81 to 3.

Dart was formally recognized for his work promoting sports for Japanese people with disabilities, as well as the employment of those individuals. He received personal congratulations from the then-Crown Prince Akihito and Princess Michiko (now emperor and empress). Dart was one of the first private sector Americans ever to appear on the cover of the *"Time* magazine of Japan," *Shukan Asahi,* in 1965. He became known in the Japanese media as "the wheelchair president," and was labeled by one magazine as "St. Justin in the Wheel Chair." He published a book of poetry written by children with disabilities, which became the best-selling book of poetry in Japan.

Shortly after moving to Japan, Dart also met and married Fusako Mich-
ishita. They had two children, Fusako Jane and Takako Sonia; Fusako was
a "great mother to them" but she "got a bad deal when she married me at
the wrong time." Dart explained, "I got off the Gandhi track and I got on
the Donald Trump track...I told myself that I could inject social responsibility
into the system, but I found that I was conning myself and I was just doing
the ordinary thing: being flamboyant and doing photo ops, making money
by any means, drinking, and chasing women."

Dart explained that, although "off track" in some ways during his time
running Japan Tupperware, "I learned a lot of things I never would have
learned any other way...there's no free lunch; work hard and sweat eighteen
hours per day; Friday comes and you have to meet the payroll...you gotta
get along with people — and the buck stops here." For example, one day
when he entered the front office of Japan Tupperware at 7:00 A.M., he found
the floor littered with papers. He started wheeling around the area, picking
up the papers. The receptionist came in and was horrified, exclaiming, "Mr.
President! You can't do that! Let me do that. It's not your job." But Dart said,
"That is my job; if I can't convince the janitor or somebody else to do it, I'd
damn well better do it myself."

Most importantly during this time, Dart hired, and grew to deeply appreciate, Yoshiko Saji, a woman he would later describe as "the greatest human
being I have ever known, because she actually lives the great traditional
principles of humanity." Dart said, "I fell in love with her, although I was
already married. It was a tremendous scandal." Justin Dart, Jr. and Yoshiko
Saji would later marry, but Dart emphasized that, "to call it a marriage, that's
a minor aspect [of the relationship]. We're partners, comrades-soldiers — it's
much, much more than a love affair." Mrs. Dart (Yoshiko) added that they
are "comrades in the struggle for a better universe."

*"Did you know she was the first woman in the history of her village to ever
graduate from a university?"*   Yoshiko Dart has said that when she was
young, she lived "a primitive life" that "to me is beautiful." She was born
and grew up during wartime when food was scarce. Although her family
members were not farmers (her father worked for the post office), they lived
on a farm and assisted with planting and harvesting rice, wheat, barley, and
sweet potatoes; they also fished in the local river. Her family lived in a house
with a bare lightbulb for illumination, and a candle lantern in the bathroom,
which had no flush toilet. They had to empty the country toilet themselves,
scoop by scoop, and bury its contents in a big hole in a field. Water had to
be pumped, and they heated bath water over a wood fire which sometimes
"smoked up" the house. Yoshiko remembers washing clothes in the river
stream even in the winter, without gloves, when her hands became cold and
numb. She would hang the clothes on bamboo poles to dry, and they would
freeze in place. Yoshiko's father was an alcoholic who had short periods of
sobriety, "but then drank again until so sick he threw up," often losing
consciousness. Yoshiko tended to be the caretaker of her family, including

her younger sisters. When Yoshiko was in junior high school, she took a year off from school to care for her mother, who had developed heart failure. Her mother died when Yoshiko was thirteen years old; Yoshiko was the head of her family at that tender age. Yoshiko has recently said that, although not by choice, "All these so-called hardships have benefited me...and helped me through all kinds of [later] hardships and psychological turmoils...I just don't give up." She noted that "Justin appreciates this."

When asked how she came to be the first woman in her village to go to a four-year university, Yoshiko recalled that during the 1950s, the American ambassador to Japan was a Harvard professor who had married a Japanese woman. Yoshiko said she wished she could be like this woman, because "America was like a God to us, after we lost the war." She wanted to become an "international-minded person," getting a job in an international company. During this time, she had a good English teacher in junior high school, one who "was tough, and cared about the students' success." That teacher was also a coach for volleyball (in which Yoshiko participated), and partly because of the teacher's involvement with sports, English became fashionable in that school. They had no television, but Yoshiko listened to the radio at a certain time each day to hear more English. When it came time to take entrance exams to get into high school, young Yoshiko had the highest overall score, and the highest score in English. During high school, she attended Bible study with an American missionary after school; she said that this missionary exposed her to "the good part of American culture." She was encouraged to go to Aoyama Gakuin, a very prestigious university in Tokyo, where there were lots of American teachers. Yoshiko's high scores on the entrance exam earned her a place in the university, as well as a room in the exclusive dormitory, housing only twenty freshmen. She explained that ninety percent of those students got in because of their connections (parents who were politicians, doctors, bank presidents, etc.), but "two of us got in because of test results." Yoshiko said she thrived on the exchange of ideas at the university, and "That's how I went from mountain country village to Tokyo."

In 1963, Yoshiko read a tiny advertisement in Japan's leading newspaper, about a company she'd never heard of. The ad stated that Japan Tupperware was "seeking ladies who are very positive and result-oriented people." The orientation meeting was in the most fashionable hotel in Tokyo, where Yoshiko had never been. She thought, "I can lose nothing, so let's go and see." While waiting for the orientation to begin, she saw a man in a wheelchair; it was the first time she'd seen anyone who was active in society using a wheelchair. It turned out that this man was Justin Dart, Jr., the president of Japan Tupperware, who told the assembled women, "We are going to try a new thing — we need you. The company will succeed or fail, depending on you." Yoshiko thought, "This is different from an ordinary company!" She decided to work for the company, and within the first week, became the number-one salesperson. Higher sales were rewarded with bigger commissions. She remembered, "Everything was so new, and depended on *our* ability!" Dart quickly asked her to become a manager. She recalled, "He instantly recognized the successes of people and promoted them. He provided servants and cars for the women staying in Tokyo, so they could focus on sales." Before long, Yoshiko was a regional supervisor, traveling by airplane and bullet-train (which was "rare for a young lady") throughout half of Japan, regularly returning to Tokyo to train young managers. "I could test my ability by doing things I wanted to do," she recalled, "which was not the norm in Japan at the time."

Because Yoshiko had a boyfriend living in Australia, Justin Dart assisted her in getting a position with Australia Tupperware. In time, Yoshiko came to believe that a marriage with that boyfriend would not work out. Dart called her, explaining that Japan Tupperware was growing so fast, he really needed good people to run it. If there was to be no marriage to the Australian boyfriend, would she please come back to Japan? Yoshiko asked, "When do you want me to come back?" He replied, "Yesterday." She thought, "Anybody interested in my ability that much — I will take advantage of that!" Within two days, she was back in Japan, and Justin Dart greeted her with a bouquet of red carnations. She was touched by this gesture. Yoshiko Saji became Justin Dart's right-hand colleague, travelling around the country with Dart and the "wheelchair boys" (basketball athletes). She was initially "violently opposed" to marrying Dart, because as Dart admitted, "There was nothing wrong with the lady I was married to. I hurt her." However, Dart and Saji, "comrades in the struggle for a better universe," eventually married in 1968, and have continued to move forward together for more than thirty years. Dart has noted, with a smile, "Ann Landers would hate this story, because usually 'the other woman' ends up in disaster."

Although Japan Tupperware was extremely successful, international Tupperware leadership was not pleased with some of Justin Dart, Jr.'s unconventional tactics, and he was ordered to better conform to corporate policy. They were not pleased with his use of national television exposure, his wheelchair donation program, or his programs to train and employ people with disabilities. Although his father, Justin Dart, Sr., privately agreed with his son's policies, he formally supported the position of the leaders working for him, and ordered Dart, Jr. to comply with his boss' mandates. Instead, Dart, Jr. resigned. He later called this action "one big mistake" that "really hurt my father."

Dart's success with Japan Tupperware did *not* land him another top-level job. Although he launched a job search, he was not offered a single interview. He then made a "not-well-researched decision," and borrowed money to start DartCard, a company selling greeting cards, with part of the proceeds dedicated to assisting people with disabilities. Although DartCard became the largest card company in Japan, Dart said "There wasn't much money in it."

In 1996, because DartCard was known as a corporate sponsor of disability causes, Dart decided to go to Vietnam, to investigate the situation in Saigon of people with disabilities. Appreciating the opportunity for publicity,

Dart's goal was to make a report to Rehabilitation International, which was about to have its World Congress in Germany. Dart took with him a professional photographer and two other assistants, Yoshiko Saji and Naoki Kurisu, a wheelchair user with paraplegia. They visited different institutions that dealt with people who had disabilities, where they took pictures and made notes. Everywhere they went, they found a "rough situation." They regularly heard artillery fire in the suburbs at night and saw the accompanying flashes of light. At some hospitals, they found two or three people in one bed, and some on the floor. Dart recalled, "There was one fellow half burned up, sitting on a window sill. You couldn't tell from looking at him — was he alive or dead?" They met a woman who had become paraplegic from a land-mine injury, and was about to be discharged. They asked her physician, "What will she do now?" The doctor responded, "She will go back to her village, and in two months she will die." There was no doctor there to provide follow-up medical care for her, and her family would probably not focus their efforts on getting her the services she would need. The doctor continued, "We do the best we can..."

"This is evil, and you are part of it."   Dart and his assistants visited an institution for children who had contracted polio. They found "a concentration camp," a giant building with a tin roof and a concrete floor. Dart described the atrocious scene: "The floor of the whole place was covered with children ages four to ten, with bloated stomachs and matchstick limbs...They were starving to death and lying in their own urine and feces, covered with flies." Dart continued, "A little girl reached up to me and looked into my eyes. I automatically took her hand and my photographer took pictures. She had the most serene look I have ever seen — and it penetrated to the deepest part of my consciousness...I thought, 'Here is a human being looking for God, looking for a miraculous solution, and instead she has found a counterfeit saint doing a photo op.' I was engulfed by the devastating perception that I have met real evil, and I am part of it...that scene is burned forever in my soul." Dart returned to his hotel, got drunk, and got sick. "And then it came to me," he said, "I could not live with myself if I didn't make an effort to do something about this." He turned to Yoshiko and said, "We cannot go on as we have been. Our lives have got to mean something. We have got to get into this fight and stop this evil."

Later, Dart met the woman who was in charge of that institution; she was wearing expensive silk and large diamonds at a fundraiser for her "wonderful" charity. Dart noted that "She was wearing ten times as much money as the whole institution cost." He suspected that the money raised actually went to her own personal use, not to meeting the needs of the children under her care. Mentally comparing her extravagant attire to the condition of the children dying on the concrete floor, Dart was speechless with horror.

Dart's report to the World Conference of Rehabilitation International was "a scathing record of atrocity, but was largely ignored by the rehabilitation establishment." There were no changes in the lives of people with disabilities in Vietnam. What did change was Dart's attitude and his perspective on life. He asked himself, "What have I been doing that got me into this situation? Where did I get off the track? Where is the track?" He noted, "I have met the enemy and it is me." He recognized that he "was drinking too much already, and had a lot of other problems." He had "made every fashionable mistake — alcohol, prescription drugs, womanizing, divorces, bad mouthing, big mouthing, bad parenting and outrageous self-advertising." He had "thought business consisted of squeezing every possible penny out of everyone." Mostly, he said, "I [had] blamed my problems and the problems of society on others." He knew that to get back on track, he needed to find his own real truth and to make a serious effort to live it.

Dart then terminated his business interests, finalized a divorce from his second wife, and married Yoshiko. Justin and Yoshiko moved to a small apartment house in the mountains in Matsumoto, Nagano-ken, Japan. Yoshiko remembered, "We didn't have much money. We ate horsemeat and whalemeat as a luxury. Justin sat on the wooden floor and cut up cabbages, onions, and carrots; that was our main source of energy. Ramen noodles for lunch were luxurious food...Japanese newspaper ads were printed on one side, and were blank on the other. We cut up the papers and used the blank sides as writing paper. We also cut up newspaper for toilet paper...It snowed a lot. We put straw rope around the wheels on the wheelchair to go out. We would wheel/walk several miles from the apartment to catch the train to go to Tokyo or other cities. Justin carried a large suitcase on the wheelchair, and could hardly see over it...We used the resources we had." During that time, Justin Dart struggled with his addictions, read history and philosophy, and corresponded with activists around the world, including poets such as Allen Ginsberg. Around this time, Dart gave back the Distinguished Alumnus Award he had received from the University of Texas, saying, "No student should follow my life." He expressed pride in returning the award; for him, this was an act of conscience. He later noted, "I may be the only ex-distinguished alumnus of any university in the United States!"

Seeking a place of reflection, the Darts then moved to a more remote region of the mountains. They rode the steam train that went highest into the mountains. In Kai Oizumi, Yamanashi-ken, they encountered a farmer who said he had an abandoned place that was "so rough" he couldn't charge them to live there, but if they taught him English, they could stay there for free. Snow and wind came through the cracks in the walls, but the Darts "fixed it into a livable place," according to Yoshiko. In this remote home, the Darts had no indoor plumbing, no central heat, nor a telephone. They had no car, but then again, if they had acquired one, there was no paved road on which to drive. Justin recalled, "In the winter Yoshiko had to hammer the ice off the pipes every day, and the snow would blow up your ass from the hole-in-the-floor country toilet." Still, Yoshiko said, this retreat home was exactly what Justin was seeking, and "he really liked it." The Darts spent six years in retreat in the mountains.

"*I am the problem. I am — all humans are — addicted to primitive self-defeating stereotypes, killing each other to gain money, power, and prestige.*" During his time in the mountains, Justin said, "I looked hard at my life...I began to truly experiment with my truth. It came as a profound shock to understand that I was the problem, that I was the solution, that I am responsible for myself, and for all the problems, for all the solutions of society. Because I am society. I am the government. I am the difference — the only difference. Only when I change will society and government change. The responsibility is mine..." His initial reaction to this insight was euphoria. With this tremendous understanding, he would be able to overcome his own addictions and stereotypes, and become a model of perfection, inspiring others..."I can see the Nobel Prize now!" he thought.

In retrospect, Dart said recently, "I couldn't have been more wrong. I soon discovered that the addictions of millennia would only be overcome by painful lifetimes of struggle." Dart had some powerful addictions to overcome. Given his success-oriented family background, he was particularly addicted to symbols of power and prestige. Yoshiko explained that when he was on the cover of *Shukan Asahi* (the *Time* magazine of Japan), he posed smoking a cigar, because he thought it made him look "like a big shot," even though he didn't really smoke at the time. While married, he had a high-class geisha girlfriend, "because high-class businessmen had them." He lived in a fancy atmosphere, "with excellent taste." He drank "lots of whiskey," although "only at night — one bottle straight per night." Yoshiko, accustomed to her father's alcoholism, said that "Justin wasn't violent, but it wasn't a beautiful scene in the middle of the nights."

Unfortunately, even with his magnificent insight, Justin Dart found his addictions difficult to eradicate. He recently explained, "Just knowing I had these addictions didn't give me the power to eliminate them. I'm still struggling." When he came to the shocking realization that his struggle to overcome addictions would be ongoing, especially addictions to stereotypical symbols of power and prestige, he became ill and depressed. He retreated further into the abuse of alcohol and prescription drugs.

Justin Dart repeatedly experienced what he and Yoshiko called "sky-rocket times," when he would pour all of his energy and excitement into one "brilliant" thing after another, and then crash back to earth. Justin explained, "I'm just a passionate person, and I've always had problems, including depression. I'm passionate about my goals, including some that were not that intelligent (the 'Donald Trump syndrome')." With Yoshiko's support, at their mountain retreat, he made great progress in facing his addictions. He began to defeat his alcoholism and addiction to prescription drugs, and to make progress in overcoming his addiction to the stereotypes of power and prestige. His "skyrocket times" gradually faded away. Yet, he still confronts addiction. He recently asserted, "While the alcohol and drugs are gone, I still struggle with power and prestige. Anybody who says they don't have these passions is lying to you...If I make five yards of progress against a one-mile addiction, that's a big deal."

In addition to dealing with addictions, Justin said, "I began to understand the power of love. I'm not talking about 'have-a-nice-day' love, or love
that controls. I'm talking about the kind of love that empowers people to
take over their own lives, to be winners by their own efforts and their own
values...This is the kind of love that has empowered our greatest leaders
and their movements, Abraham, Jesus, Buddha, Muhammad, Gandhi, Martin Luther King..." The Darts began to look more closely at how to lovingly

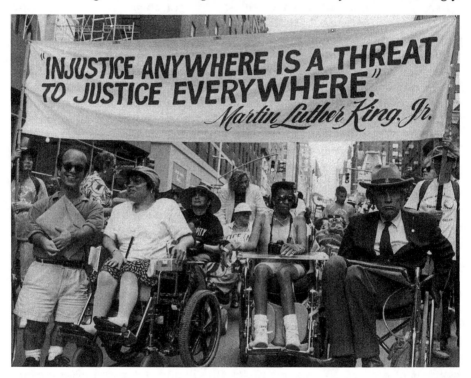

empower people. Yoshiko recalled, "Justin was always interested in under-
dog-type people. Before we met, he had helped some girl in Mexico to
become a movie star...When we lived in the mountains, one lady who used
to be an employee of DartCard helped us with some typing, and we helped
her to become more independent. She was reading lots of books. Then Justin
had an idea: why not help students who had failed entrance exams get into
universities?" The Darts went into the countryside and found a young girl
whose dream was to go to the United States and become a nurse. She came
to live with them; Justin taught her English and how to study at an American
college. She was accepted into a college in Texas, and later went to another
college in Kentucky to study nursing. "She was so successful," Yoshiko said,
"Her cousins wanted to come into our life." Through word of mouth, church
members, siblings, and others found out about the Dart's "life-quality training program." Over the past thirty years, the Darts have had eighty foster
daughters and two foster sons living with them, for periods of time ranging

from six months to several years. At one time, they had eleven trainees living with them in the small mountain farmhouse in Japan. "That was too many," sighed Yoshiko.

Around the time Justin Dart was feeling more confident about his new philosophy, making significant progress in defeating alcoholism and addiction to prescription drugs, and experiencing success with empowering young people, he was called back to the United States. His grandmother had passed away, and then his mother committed suicide. He needed to go to Seattle to attend to several matters, including access to a trust fund, which was released upon his mother's death.

"Stigma..."   Dart said, "My mother, who was very wealthy, an award-winning author published by Alfred Knopf, who looked like a movie star, who had famous boyfriends like Adlai Stevenson, killed herself." He explained that she didn't seek any treatment for depression "because she was afraid of the stigma" associated with mental illness. Later, Justin's brother, Peter Dart, also struggled with disability-related stigma. He was a successful man, an Air Force jet pilot, with a graduate degree in engineering, a "trophy wife," children, and lots of money. However, he contracted polio, and "didn't want to accept his disability," according to Justin. "He didn't want help, he wanted a cure." Peter would "get angry" with Justin, because Justin used a wheelchair instead of trying to walk. Peter, strapped in leg braces, "fell down some steps and suffered a severe brain injury, a more serious disability, because of it," explained Justin. As Peter continued "taking more falls, pretending he wasn't disabled," his family urged him to seek to rehabilitation services, and to use a wheelchair. Then they actually bought him a wheelchair, and his eldest son said to him, "Dad, we love you; we don't want you to hurt yourself. Please use this [wheelchair]." Peter Dart looked at the chair and said, "I'd rather be dead." Two days later, he was dead. Ironically, Justin said, "I thought I had convinced him to go to the Houston Independent Living Center. When I called his secretary to set up the appointment details, she said, 'He died last night.' I felt guilty...when I was out preaching to the world about empowerment and independence, my own brother needed my attention, didn't get it, and died...I was too late." At first, Justin Dart told himself that there wasn't much he could have done, because his brother had so strongly rejected him. But then he said to himself, "Bullshit, Justin: You could have reached out," even though "it wasn't real comfortable."

Justin Dart bought a modest house in Seattle, and decorated it with artwork he had begun to collect. He said the house was part of "a government experiment designed to allow lower-income people to buy houses." He and Yoshiko moved their life-quality training program to this home, and several Japanese girls came to live there. However, Justin didn't find any people in Seattle who were excited about his philosophy and ideas about empowerment. He decided that the best way to spread his philosophical revolution was to connect with the disability rights movement. In 1978, the

Darts and their foster family moved to Austin, Texas, where Justin became involved with the local disability rights group, MIGHT. He met experienced leaders in the movement, including Ed Roberts and Judy Heumann, who Dart said "took me to kindergarten" in terms of disability rights. Dart co-founded an independent living center in Austin and became active in local politics and fundraising activities. He then served in five gubernatorial appointments related to disability policy in the state of Texas. In 1981, when Ronald Reagan was the newly elected president of the United States and was replacing all of the members of the National Council on Disability, Justin Dart, Jr. was a prominent figure in Texas politics. That, and probably Dart's father's reputation as leader of Reagan's informal "kitchen cabinet" of powerful advisors, earned him an appointment as vice chair of the Council. Dart said, "I don't know if my father was in favor of my appointment, but I do know that if he was specifically opposed to it, I would not have been offered the position."

"My father was a famous politician who never held office."   Justin Dart, Jr. once asked his father, "How do you get this outstanding political power?" Justin Dart, Sr. replied to his son, "Everybody goes to the White House and tells the president what they want...I go there, and never tell him what I want; I ask him what I can do — what do *they* want? And then I do it. And then they pay attention." Justin Dart, Jr. has described his father as "a very secure and self-disciplined person," and added, "Did you know that he also was awarded a Presidential Medal of Freedom?" Dart explained, "He perceived a great threat to democracy from the communists. Many people said that trying to bring down the 'evil empire' was a hopeless cause, but he spent an enormous amount of money and energy convincing people around the world to fight this fight." Dart summarized with pride, "My father was a quarterback, or coach of a worldwide effort to bring down the Soviet police state." He added, "We were probably the first father/son pair to win the Freedom award...he won it from an administration on the far right, and I won it from one on the left."

In his appointment to the National Council on Disability (NCD — at that time, it was called the National Council on the Handicapped), Justin Dart, Jr. found great opportunities to channel his passion for advocacy. With the full support of NCD chair, Joe Dusenbury, Dart traveled to each of the fifty states to involve local disability-rights leaders in the creation of a national policy for people with disabilities. When the resulting policy document was drafted, Dart introduced it to the NCD. He recalled that one of the NCD members said, "This is a nice thing, Justin, but we got to get some of these radical-rights proposals [like the forerunner of the ADA] out of here." Other members of the Reagan-appointed, heavily conservative council "sort of nodded." Then, according to Dart, "Joe Dusenbury stood up to full height and let some silence lapse, very dramatic. He picked up the document and he said, 'Ladies and gentlemen, this document was written by the

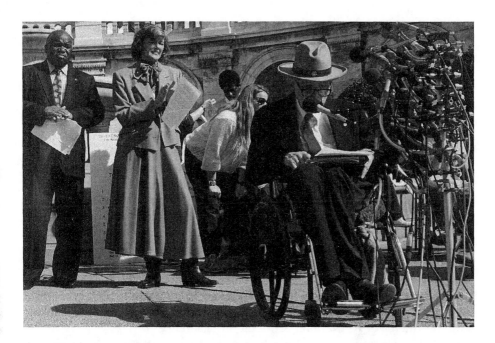

disabled people of the United States. I want to hear a motion to approve this document and I don't want you to change a single word.' There was a silence, and then there was a motion to approve, and the document was approved without change. It was followed by a signed endorsement by President Reagan. And this is one of the reasons Joe Dusenbury lost that job as chairman of the National Council, the only significant defeat in his life, because he took that and other stands on principle."

"Real life equality occurs only through the advocacy and eternal vigilance of those who seek it."   In 1986, Dart recalled, members of the NCD came to the conclusion that disability discrimination was distinctive, and required a separate civil rights law. Under the leadership of Chairperson Sandra Parrino, Director Lex Frieden, and disability rights attorney Bob Burgdorf, the Americans with Disabilities Act (ADA) became the foremost recommendation of the Council's report, *Toward Independence*. The White House called, and said, "What were you folks thinking about with this civil rights thing? The president won't touch it with a ten-foot pole. Take it out." Director Frieden and Dart decided to take a stand instead of trying to negotiate to keep the controversial recommendation. Dart met with the assistant attorney general for civil rights, Bradford Reynolds. He asserted, "Bradford, I do not believe Ronald Reagan wants to go down in history as the president who opposed keeping the promise of the Declaration of Independence to 35 million Americans with disabilities." After a lapse of silence, Reynolds responded, "Justin, the president is not going to oppose your report, he is going to support it in writing." (Reagan did, indeed, provide that written support.)

Also in 1986, Reagan appointed Justin Dart, Jr. to head the Rehabilitation Services Administration (RSA). At the time Dart accepted the appointment, the RSA was a three-billion-dollar agency with a reputation for inefficiency and paternalism. Dart ordered a study of how long it took, on average, to initiate services for vocational rehabilitation clients with disabilities. He was appalled to find that the average client coming into one of those offices would have to wait 5.4 months before receiving his or her first services. Dart has said that rehabilitation counselors *should* be more like coaches, whose job is to empower their clients. Like coaches, the counselors should strive to bring out the very best in all of their clients, "so they will be bigger stars than he [or she] is." In 1987, Dart read a "statement of conscience" to a packed Congressional hearing. He told the assembled members, "We are confronted by a vast, inflexible federal system which, like the society it represents, still contains a significant proportion of individuals who have not yet overcome obsolete, paternalistic attitudes about disability..." Within days, Dart was asked to resign from the RSA. Dart refused to "trash" in the media President Reagan or his more immediate supervisor, Madeleine Will, for the circumstances surrounding his resignation. That fact, in addition to a great amount of support expressed for him by the disability community, resulted in his reappointment to the National Council on Disability.

In 1988, Dart was named co-chair of the newly created Congressional Task Force on the Rights and Empowerment of Americans with Disabilities. This group was charged with the task of gathering information and making recommendations to Congress regarding the proposed ADA. Dart appointed a distinguished and diverse group of advocates to his panel, with the intention of unifying fragmented elements of the disability community, to powerfully support the ADA. He included not only the traditionally represented individuals with physical or sensory disabilities, but also advocates with psychiatric disabilities or mental retardation. Some individuals expressed concern that "we should not have representatives of people with AIDS; people with AIDS will die." Dart responded emphatically, "Of course they will die; so will you and I. We are not into perpetuating paternalism." He appointed two people with AIDS to the task force.

The Task Force was given no public funds to carry out its mission, but between 1988 and 1990, Dart personally chaired sixty-three public forums across the country, including at least one in every state, plus Guam and Puerto Rico. Utilizing his own resources and contributions by local disability rights advocates, he reached more than 30,000 people, and filed thousands of petitions and statements about disability discrimination, which were presented by the carton to Congress.

In 1989, President George Bush appointed Dart to chair the President's Committee on Employment of People with Disabilities. Dart was accused of changing the focus of the committee from employment to disability rights, to which he replied, "I plead guilty. No transportation, no health care, no education; no civil rights, no jobs." Dart's passion was focused on passage of the ADA. In pursuit of this goal, he visited each state between four and twenty times, meeting with groups numbering from three individuals to six thousand. In support of this goal, he met with anybody he could, from residents of nursing homes to the president of the United States. He visited every congressional office, many of them several times. "Often," he recalled, "I would roll into a congressperson's office in my wheelchair, and before I said anything I would be greeted by, 'Yes, we know — ADA, no weakening amendments." "I became a symbol," he said. When it comes to talking with politicians, he noted, "I am more excessive than most."

"Some people say I'm a zealot... I am an extremist, a zealot." Justin Dart, Jr. has accepted the label "zealot", the "positive connotation of an extremist," with pride. Dart gave the following example of his zealousness. One evening when he was in Oklahoma City, he was told that President Bush wanted to meet with him the next morning in Washington, D.C. Dart made reservations for a flight back to D.C., but when the van, which was inaccessible, took him out to the airplane, there was nobody there to lift him out of the van seat, except the "ancient" van driver. The driver tried to lift Dart out of his seat, but he slipped, and Dart's leg got caught under the seat. The driver then dropped Dart, breaking his trapped leg. Still, Dart got into the plane, flew to D.C., met with the president, flew back, gave his scheduled talk in Oklahoma City, and then continued on his circuit of speaking engagements. Dart said that he never did see a doctor to treat the broken bone; "the leg healed by itself." When asked whether he had felt pain in the leg, he replied, "Of course!" and explained that the day one breaks a bone is *not* the most painful day — "it gets a lot worse a few days later." Still, he said with pride, "That's the definition of a zealot."

"This is the first declaration of equality for people with disabilities around the world." In 1990, Congress passed the Americans with Disabilities Act. Dart explained the significance and importance of this landmark legislation: "I consider its passage to be one of the great moral and political miracles in the history of democracy. A ragtag hodgepodge of advocates with disabilities, families, and service providers, who had never completely agreed on anything before, joined together with a few far-sighted members of the older civil rights movement, business, the Congress and the Administration to defeat the richest, most powerful lobbies in the nation. It is a story to rival the creation of the Declaration of Independence and the victory of the American Revolution." On July 26, 1990, Justin Dart, Jr. appeared on the dais with President George Bush while the president signed the Americans with Disabilities Act; Bush gave Dart the first pen he used to sign the law. Despite blazing heat and oppressive humidity that day, Dart said that moving the ADA signing ceremony indoors "was inconceivable; the biggest room in the White House wouldn't hold more than three hundred...Three thousand people gathered on the south lawn of the White House to witness this event, the largest attendance at any signing ceremony in the history of the United States."

When asked at the time about the heat and humidity, Dart replied, "I'd go through a lot more than that for this day!"

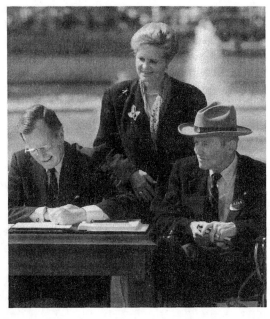

Until 1993, Dart continued to serve as chair of the President's Committee on Employment of People with Disabilities, focusing on implementation of the employment provisions of the ADA. He met with leaders of the business and disability communities, urging "full and harmonious compliance with the ADA, with minimal litigation and expense, and maximum employment for people with disabilities and profit for business." However, Dart noticed with concern that the ADA would not be of much use in securing access to affordable health care for people with disabilities. In October 1993, Justin Dart resigned his position as chair of the President's Committee, vowing to become a "full-time citizen soldier for justice." His first mission in that role was the promotion of universal access to health care as a fundamental right of every American.

"We are willing to die for our country, but not for our insurance companies." Dart campaigned for health care reform across the country, sometimes speaking on the same platform as President Bill Clinton, Vice President Al Gore, or First Lady Hillary Clinton. He also made a dramatic gesture to emphasize a point, saying that he had examined his conscience and realized "that I have not risked enough. I have not fought enough. I have not loved enough. I have not spent enough. There will be no replacement of the ancient car. No speeches in Europe. There will be more confrontation, more dollars, and hours invested in justice...Today I will cancel my health care insurance. I was able to have it only because I was once a federal employee. Probably it cannot be replaced. My conscience will no longer allow me to pay an immorally high premium, to contribute $16,152.24 per year to full-page insurance-industry ads in the *Washington Post*, justifying a system that is oppressing our people. I will give that money and more to buy our own ad...Some very smart people have said this is a dumb thing to do — a very high risk. Maybe so. Sometimes you act from the heart and the soul." Dart later noted, that once cancelled, this policy indeed could not be replaced, because of his disability.

"Get into politics as if your life depended on it. It does."   After the rise of the political far right in the 1994 elections, Justin Dart and disability rights advocates, Fred Fay and Becky Ogle, formed "Justice for All," an organization dedicated to mobilizing grassroots advocacy for issues impacting people with disabilities. Dart watched his beloved Republican party not only defeat attempts to reform health care in America, but in general move toward "a tragic politics of retreat." Dart believed this radical swing, away from a model of empowerment, would "condemn millions of Americans with disabilities to unemployment, welfare, and charity; to isolation and institutions in backrooms; to poor health, and for many, to early death." Loyal to the Republican party, Dart had historically taken the lead in organizing people with disabilities in support of Ronald Reagan's and George Bush's presidential campaigns. He had served in multiple posts appointed by Republican presidents. However, in 1996, he saw his party's presidential candidate, Bob Dole, endorse the agenda of the "new Republican politics of retreat." Dart made an agonizingly difficult decision. First in a press conference, and again from the stage of the Democratic National Convention in Chicago, he declared: "I am a Republican. I have a message for Bob Dole. Senator, I respect you. I have supported you. I love you. But I love the American dream more. I have made a painful decision of conscience. In 1996, I am a Republican for Clinton." Dart then set out to galvanize people with disabilities into taking political action for the candidates of their own choice. Leaders of the disability community made these decisions: approximately 2500 chose to publicly campaign for Bill Clinton; around two hundred chose to support the campaign of Bob Dole. After the final vote counts were tallied, the re-elected President Clinton recognized that "Justin Dart went to every state to organize Americans with disabilities for the Clinton-Gore campaign. That's one reason we won some of those states." Dart added, "the final vote counts revealed that Americans with disabilities had given a record 46-point margin to Bill Clinton." Dart predicted that in the future, people with disabilities will be "one of the most powerful voting constituencies."

"People with disabilities have no million-dollar political action committees. Yoshiko and I have tried our best to be a little PAC for empowerment, contributing to members of both parties who support people with disabilities." Even after the 1996 election, Justin and Yoshiko Dart focused their energies and financial resources in ways they believed would have a significant political impact. They ran this PAC for empowerment out of their home, a small two-bedroom apartment in Washington, D.C. Their apartment served as their residence and office, and as always, as a location for the life-quality training program to empower their foster children. Justin explained, "We've been doing experiments in empowerment for thirty years. It works." Yoshiko added, "It's very rewarding." She continued, "All the people who went through the program are truly independent...all of them went on to do something exceeding their initial dreams...That's the best present you can give." She noted that over the years, the Darts had only one foster child that they "shipped back home." She explained, "Only people who want to be part of our program are here. Responsibility is a training, "which is learned through activities such as handling telephone calls, mending, grocery shopping, preparing expense reports, etc." Yoshiko added that, "Now they all learn computer skills, too." She said that Justin has the drive to motivate and push the foster children, to "remind them of their own goals." "We know they make mistakes," she said, but that is part of how they learn. At times, it must have been somewhat amusing for political movers and shakers in the nation's capitol to reach a receptionist-in-training. *"Yes, Senator, and how do you spell your name? Okay, K-E-N-N-..."* "Give me that phone!" exclaimed Dart. Later, he heard, *"Mr. Dart, a president wants to talk to you."* "Which president is it?" *"President Reagan."*

Among the eighty-two foster children the Darts have empowered over the years are people with severe psychoses and other psychiatric disabilities, physical disabilities, developmental disabilities, learning disabilities, sensory disabilities, and other challenges. Many of them had financial, educational, family, and other personal problems. The Darts focused on giving these young people the tools they needed to empower themselves, transcending stereotypes, and gaining confidence in their abilities. The Darts have provided personal and career counseling, as well as financial assistance, to their foster children, but mostly they described their role as that of being the empowering "coaches" of these young people. Yoshiko explained, "I want them to become better than I am in many ways, and if they can teach their children to be better than they do, the world will become a better place."

"Another stereotype we have to fight against is the idea that we will live forever." In December of 1997, Justin Dart was experiencing the effects of post-polio syndrome, as well as numerous additional health problems. He was hospitalized at Georgetown Medical Center with a diagnosis of massive congestive heart failure. According to Dart, his doctors had "pretty well exhausted the resources of science," including surgical insertion of a pacemaker to regulate his heartbeat. They admitted to Dart that they had not been able to restore his heart to a non-life-threatening condition, and they wanted him to remain in the hospital. He thanked them for saving his life, and recognized that they were "world-class professional people" who "meant well." However, he continued, "...they are underfunded and understaffed. Their obsolete hospital, system, and attitudes are significantly hostile to people with disabilities. I felt like a subhuman — a laboratory rat in a cage." After eight days in the hospital, Dart decided, "against the advice of several doctors...to continue my life and my fight for my life in my home." He explained, "Here I am surrounded by people I love. Here I am in command of my life. Here I am senior partner in my own health care. Here I can continue my politics of freedom." He recognized the potential cost, but emphasized the goals of his decision: "I was told that I might not live as long. Maybe not. This is a matter of principle...This is my insistence to live free as human beings were meant to live...This is my protest against a system

that coerces millions of people with and without disabilities to be caged in hospitals, nursing homes, and other oppressive settings." Dart added his heartfelt appeal: "Let us unite in a revolution to eliminate primitive practices and stereotypes, and to establish a culture that focuses the full force of science and democracy on the systematic empowerment of every person to live his or her God given potential. No soldier ever died in a better cause."

Dart did return to his home, with the assistance of a personal care attendant "and the support of the magnificent hospice organization in [Washington] D.C." Here, he was again surrounded by people he loved, in familiar surroundings. He could look over the apartment walls still crowded with photographs and posters of people and events important in his advocacy struggles over the years; he was living among his books about people he respected, such as Abraham Lincoln and Mohandas Gandhi. Among the books on one side of his room was a children's book by Watty Piper, entitled *The Little Engine That Could.* Hanging over Dart's desk was a poem that had originally hung in his grandfather's living room:

> *Outwitted*
> By Edwin Markham
>
> He drew a circle that shut me out —
> Heretic, rebel, a thing to flout.
> But love and I had the wit to win:
> We drew a circle that took him in!

"Injustice anywhere is a threat to justice everywhere."   This quote, attributed to Martin Luther King, Jr., is written across a large banner that Justin and Yoshiko Dart have often carried in demonstrations. On Martin Luther King's birthday, in January of 1998, President Clinton presented Justin Dart, Jr. with the Medal of Freedom. Clinton said,

> Justin Dart literally opened the doors of opportunities to millions of our citizens by securing passage of one of the nation's landmark civil rights laws: The Americans with Disabilities Act...At the University of Houston, he led bold efforts to promote integration. He went on to become, in his own words, "a full-time soldier in the trenches of justice," touring every state in the nation to elevate disability rights to the mainstream of political discourse. He once said, "Life is not a game that requires losers." He has given millions a chance to win. He has also been my guide in understanding the needs of disabled Americans. And every time I see him, he reminds me of the power of heart and will. I don't know that I've ever known a braver person.

When he presented the medal to Dart, President Clinton hugged him and said, "I love you," using the words Dart so often said to others. After Dart came down from the stage, he took off the medal and placed it on Yoshiko, who he has credited with "way over half of everything we've done together." Later, Yoshiko said, "I got very emotional...We have lived together and fought for justice together. He really showed his love and respect and appreciation to me in that way. And not just as his wife, but as a comrade and soldier together in the struggle." Justin proclaimed to everyone in the disability rights movement: "This is your medal. I am so proud to be one of you. I will fight at your side until the last breath."

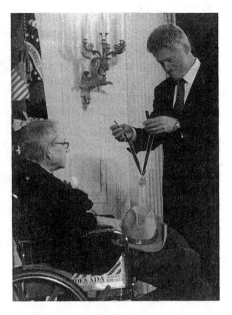

"I won't change history single-handedly, but maybe I can plant a few seeds of revolution that will grow." After returning home from the hospital, Dart said he was "looking up close at my mortality — stripping away things not important, one by one." Despite his physical limitations, and confined to his rented hospital bed much of the time, he continued to immerse himself in politics, to take part in demonstrations, to make public statements about important issues whenever possible, and to use his status as a recognized and respected leader, to take the revolution of empowerment to the world. These activities all became more exhausting than they had been in the past, both for Justin and for Yoshiko, who added Justin's personal-care-attendant duties to her previous responsibilities. Yet, neither Justin nor Yoshiko seemed shaken from their work by the fact that Justin "may die tonight." Comrades in the struggle for a better universe, they continued to fight to communicate the revolution of empowerment.

When asked what he would like most for people to learn from reading about his life, Justin Dart, Jr. replied, "All people, no matter how few abilities they may have, can struggle to find their personal truth, can struggle with their personal addictions, can make a big difference in society, as they change themselves. This is true for anybody. When you change yourself, you change society, because you are society." He continued, "Don't give the impression that I have won — defeated my addictions. As you see me, I struggle." *"And you expect to continue struggling?"* asked the biographer. "Right up to the last minute," Dart smiled.

chapter four

Judy Heumann

Linda R. Shaw

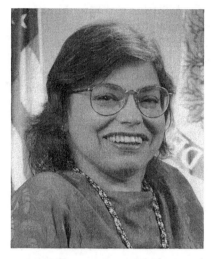

Monday morning, 8:15 A.M. — Several people are gathered upstairs in her office waiting for the conference call, and the damn elevator's out — again. Judy is exasperated. She is about to go to the office next door to call upstairs when the elevator lets out a prolonged *gri-ii-ind*, then whirs into life and lands at her floor with a final scrape and bump. After the doors slowly creak open, Judy whizzes through them, wondering if the teleconference is worth putting her life on the line by riding in this dying relic of an elevator. But she knows it is. The IDEA is under attack, and she has lots to say about that — lots.

She comes through the door and quickly sizes up the situation. The call hasn't come through yet. Whew! She waves to her colleagues, already gathered around the speaker phone at the desk in the inner office, and stops to pick up her messages. Sara hands the messages to her and says, "The top one's from Ilse. She just called again as you came in. She says it's urgent." A prickle of fear washes over her. She pushes back the little voice that insists, "It's the cancer — it's back." "You want to talk to her?" Judy glances into the office. Someone's telling a joke — some political thing, and they're all waiting for the punchline. Judy says, "Yeah, quick. Just put her on your speaker." "Ma, what is it? I've got a big meeting here in a minute." Ilse's voice always centers her — always helps her maintain her balance. Smooth and clear, her mother's voice comes through the line. "Oh, they didn't tell

1-57444-083-7/00/$0.00+$.50
© 2000 by CRC Press LLC

me! Well, I just wanted to talk to you about a situation. There's a new family that just started coming to temple, and they're getting the runaround from VR on their daughter. You should see her. She's a gorgeous girl — and smart like you. Apparently, the office is low on money and they can't do anything, but if they don't, this girl will have to drop out of school. She wants to study medicine and…" Judy looks at Sara and rolls her eyes, but can't help smiling. She knows that to her mother, not even a teleconference with the president himself would be more important than the plight of a mom whose daughter is being held back because of her disability. Just as she starts to reply, Sara signals her. Everybody's on the line except her. "Ma, I gotta go. I'll call you later and see what I can do, okay?" "Okay, Judy. See you later." She grabs the rest of the phone message slips and heads toward the door to her office. There is already a stack of them — little pink slips. Her life revolves around those little pink slips, and the phone calls — endless phone calls. Still, how many people can say they love their work? She is in her element. She heads into the meeting and slips seamlessly into place as the gathered body of government officials strains their ears and their bodies toward her speaker phone. Here goes another day.

In the beginning

Werner opened his eyes and gazed at the shadows on the ceiling from the moonlight shining through the tree by the front window. He had been lying with his eyes squeezed shut, somehow thinking he could will himself to go to sleep, but it was no use. He gave up pretending that sleep might come, and instead let his mind sift through the crazy pieces of the day. Ilse had decided to sleep at the hospital, and she had finally persuaded him to go home to sleep. His brother, Leon, could open the shop tomorrow, but Werner would still have to work. Now they would need even more money for hospital bills. Never had he experienced a feeling of the intensity he had felt today. As he gazed down at little Judy — not even two years old — he still felt wrapped in the numbness that had enveloped him upon the doctor's utterance of the dreaded diagnosis: "*polio.*" Ilse had sat down so fast and hard that he had reached out a hand to steady her, thinking she was falling. She was eight months pregnant, and her stomach was so huge that people were making jokes about her having swallowed prize-winning watermelon seeds. She shouldn't be spending the night at the hospital. But she had insisted. Judy looked so tiny — so vulnerable.

Ilse asked lots of questions, which the doctor, and then the nurse, had patiently tried to answer: "We don't know…we can't tell…we have to wait." They were unsatisfying answers to impossible questions. At the time, he had not felt angry, or sad, or really much of anything. He had just felt a sense of unreality. But later, in the hospital room, gazing down at his daughter, he felt a rush of emotion unlike any he had ever experienced. It wasn't anger, exactly; if he had analyzed it, he might have thought it had sprung from anger, but instead it was a fierce sense of determination — fierce and very personal, all wrapped up in an intense love and protectiveness toward his little girl. The feeling was almost palpable — it could almost be touched, and smelled, and breathed. It washed through his every pore, and charged his entire system with a sudden rush of adrenaline.

The only feeling he had to compare it to was the time, years ago, when he had been turned away — again — from the recruiter's desk. He had left Germany at the age of fourteen. Although the adults in his life tried to shield him from what was happening to his family in Germany, he had picked up plenty from the hushed conversations, the sad looks, the anger and despair that always seemed to accompany conversations about his kinfolk and the Jews in Germany. He hated the Nazis, and he hated the Japanese for their parts in the war. He was determined to personally strike a blow against such cruel inhumanity. Werner sized himself up in the mirror. He was only seventeen and had a schoolboy's face, and he was not very tall. Could he pass for eighteen? He practiced striding like a self-assured, fully grown man. He worked to make his voice as deep as it would go. Could he pull it off?

The recruiter laughed. "Go home," he said. "You're too young, and too short, and you aren't even a citizen." A citizen? He had not even considered that. "Go home and do some stretching exercises," the recruiters laughed. Werner left the office with a determined stride. He walked the four-and-a-half miles to the public library in about forty-five minutes, and within a few more minutes was poring over the materials the librarian had given him, which explained how to become a U.S. citizen. He studied the men he knew who appeared most "manly." How did they walk? How did they talk? He willed himself to be taller. He learned the history and the requirements for citizenship. Finally, the day came. He performed flawlessly and became a U.S. citizen. After the judge pronounced him a citizen of the United States, he headed straight to the recruiter's office. Time had passed and most of the eligible young men had already shipped off, so the recruiters were not quite as particular as they had been. He was only seventeen, but he would soon be eighteen, and he was now a citizen, after all. He had as much a right as anyone to strike a blow against the Nazis. Werner swelled with pride as he was sworn in as a member of the U.S. Marine Corps — a sense of pride that expanded and grew with time, and with his service as a member of the elite group known as Carlson's Raiders.

As determined as he had been to enlist, that was almost insignificant compared to the way he felt now. He had been alone then. Now he had Ilse to fight along with him. Then, he had been fighting for an important, yet impersonal cause. Now, he was fighting for his daughter's life. He did not know how or where to start. He knew Ilse did not know either. But he knew Ilse would be with him; Judy was her daughter, too — in some ways, even more her daughter than his. For eighteen months, Ilse had rocked her, fed her, and was with her now, even while eight months pregnant. Yes, Ilse would fight.

Ilse shifted for the hundredth time, trying to find a comfortable corner of the lumpy, hospital room chair. The relatives had all left, and she had finally persuaded Werner to go get some rest. Only by appealing to his sense of duty to work and family had she been able to convince him to go home. Eight-year-old Ricky would need someone, too, and they would need the money earned from the butcher shop that Werner owned with his brother. It wouldn't do for business to drop off now. Ilse propped her elbows on the arms of the chair and cradled her chin in her hands. What would the future hold for them now? She had been shocked when the doctor told them Judy had polio. She had looked up at Werner's stunned face. After the war, Ilse had heard plenty about shell-shock, and he looked now the way she'd pictured those people. He looked as if he just couldn't fit all the crazy little bits of life together enough to know what to do with them. She bit her lip and willed herself to stay calm and focus. There were things they would need to do, things they would need to know. She searched her mind for the questions she should ask: Will she live? Will she able to walk? What can we do? It seemed as if the only thing to do right now was to wait and to pray. Somehow, Ilse had an uneasy feeling that her life had just changed in a big way, but she couldn't say exactly how yet. She needed to know more, to understand more. Ilse tried to think — who in her wide circle of friends could help her? There was Mrs. Heinz from the PTA, whose husband was a doctor. She could call her tomorrow. She didn't know his specialty, but he'd probably know how she could get more information. It wasn't much, but it was something — something to *do*. Her thoughts were interrupted by a sharp and very insistent kick. She rubbed her stomach absently, murmuring comforting noises to the baby within. As she did so, her eyes slid toward her little daughter lying in the bed. "Hush," she said, smoothing her hands over her stomach, "Mama's here. Mama's here."

From home to school

Judy had always regarded the bang of the door as her brothers lit out of the house in the morning with mixed feelings. She liked her brothers well enough, and sort of wished she could be with them as they ran off for school with the other kids. On the other hand, she also liked the couple of minutes after her brothers had left. Every day, for just these few minutes, her mom sat still long enough to sip a cup of coffee, and Judy had her all to herself. She knew that in a few minutes, her mom would take a final swallow of the coffee, and start on her list of the million-and-one things that she seemed to find time for every day.

Today, her mom sipped her coffee and organized her day while Judy finished her cereal. She had to pick up the house before the home instruction teacher, Mrs. Wright, arrived, buy new winter boots for Ricky and Joey, bake cookies for Joey's Cub Scout meeting, place the calls she had volunteered to make for the PTA, drop off the kids at Hebrew school, take Judy to her piano lesson — and oh, yeah, remember to call the piano tuner. The piano had slowly been going out of tune. She'd tolerated it for awhile, but lately every time anyone hit that high F...well, let's just say it was finally time to invest in a tuning. Somehow, all these things would have to be scheduled, but they would have to fit around the most critical activity of the day — tonight at 7:00, she and a small group of parents were meeting with the board of education. This meeting was the culmination of months of work. Ilse had surprised herself with her ability to deal with the administrators and board members. She guessed she had somewhere acquired the "moxie" that she hadn't known she had. In the beginning, a few people seemed to listen to her, then other parents began to join her. She found herself increasingly designated as spokesperson of the group of concerned parents. She wasn't quite sure how it had happened. She only knew one thing: she was determined that Judy *would* go to school.

Ilse reflected for a moment on how things had gotten to this point. Her mind drifted back to that night when they got the diagnosis. All alone in Judy's hospital room, she had decided she would do whatever needed to be done, and that Judy would survive. She would do more than survive — if it was humanly possible to give Judy a normal life, Ilse would make it happen. She smiled to herself, and thought about how young and naive she had been. She had known nothing! Nothing about the wheelchairs, the treatments, or the exercises. Nothing about the doctors who had spouted gloom and doom and had recommended institutionalization for her daughter. Nothing about the teachers who had insisted that her little girl was too "different" to be educated in a regular school. She had taken everyone's word for it at first. They were the experts, after all; what did she know? But little by little, she came to realize that they might know a lot, but she knew Judy. She knew that Judy had a quick mind, and aside from the wheelchair, was as normal as anyone. It was clear that the home instruction teacher could not possibly give her the quality of educational and social experiences that she would need. Why was it so difficult for everyone else to see that? From her early, innocent questions, she had discovered that the school system had firm ideas about how handicapped children should be educated — ideas that did not accommodate her own parental instincts about her daughter.

For her part, Judy was pretty content with how things were. True, she didn't go to school, but she had friends in the neighborhood. She didn't think she was all that different. She played house, and knew all of the jump rope rhymes, and she was the official scorekeeper for the more physical games she couldn't play. She knew she was good at her studies — thanks to Dad and his constant history lessons. It seemed as if every time she turned around, her dad had her, or Joey, or Ricky, looking up something in the encyclopedia. She knew that encyclopedia set had cost her parents a lot of money, and could remember them buying it, one book at a time. When Judy was little, she had always thought how beautiful those volumes looked side-by-side on the shelf — all those books with their white leather bindings and softly gleaming gold letters. She was, however, kind of curious about this place called "school." The kids talked about it all the time, and it both attracted her and scared her. It would be nice to join in conversations about kids she didn't know or about various teachers, but she was okay with her little world, too. She knew her way around it pretty well, and at Brownies she got to "hang" with the kids who attended Hebrew school.

So, Judy was shocked the night her parents sat down and told her she would be going to school the next year. School! Her mother explained that the board of education had decided to designate certain schools for kids in wheelchairs. She explained that Judy would have to get up earlier, because she would have to ride the bus to her new school, which was an hour and a half away. Judy was confused. "But Mom, the school's just a couple of blocks away." "No, Judy," mom explained, "the school for handicapped kids is farther away. There's one with special classes here in Brooklyn, but that one...well, you just can't go to that one." "Special classes?," Judy asked. Was she "special," she wondered to herself? "The classes are for handicapped kids," explained her mother.

After Judy had gone to bed, Ilse told Werner about the board meeting. Werner wondered aloud what three hours of travel, to and from school, would mean to Judy. Would she be so tired from the trip that she would not be able to enjoy her family and neighborhood friends? Why would she have to be bused out of Brooklyn? Ilse's face hardened slightly as she explained that the local school superintendent considered Judy to be a "fire hazard," because of her wheelchair. "But why," wondered Werner, "could she not attend regular classes with non-handicapped kids?" Ilse explained, "They say that since she can't push her own wheelchair or walk, she will need more help than the regular teachers can provide, and they don't even want to hear about having to help her in the bathroom!" Werner sighed, and Ilse explained that she had finally conceded that this was as far as the school board would allow itself to be pushed. "It's a start, Werner," she said tiredly. Werner drew her to him and kissed her hair. "You did good," he assured her with a hug.

That night, Judy lay in bed and wondered, "What will the school be like? What will it be like to be 'special?'" Well, she had the whole summer ahead of her before that happened. Fall was a long way away, and tomorrow her aunts, uncles, and cousins were coming over for her brother's birthday. She pushed thoughts of "school" from her mind, and focused instead on the delicious and slightly superior feeling of knowing what her brother was getting for his birthday. For weeks, she had been taunting him with the fact that she knew, and he didn't. Tomorrow would be fun. By next year, she would be older, and she would manage "school" just fine. Judy drifted off to sleep, thinking about tomorrow, and the summer vacation to come.

School days

"Well," Judy thought wryly, "I guess this is 'special.'" Judy had become accustomed to the sequence of lessons and activities which school had turned out to be. Her class was called a "health conservation class," and was held in the school's basement. Her new friends in school were a variety of kids with different kinds of handicaps. Little by little, she figured out what "special" meant. It seemed to mean that you probably couldn't do much, or hope to accomplish much in life. As she learned the lay of the land at her new school, she figured out that you were written off in varying degrees, depending on how handicapped you were. If you were in a wheelchair, like she was, you were a problem. If you were in a wheelchair, and had a speech disability, that was a bigger problem. And, if you were in a wheelchair, and had a speech disability, and had some learning disabilities, that was an even bigger problem.

The confusing part was that, although her school operated on this system of logic, things were totally different at home and at camp. Her teachers seemed to think that they couldn't hold it against her if she failed to do her homework or got a "B" on a test, because she was handicapped, but her parents seemed to have missed out on this part of their own education. They continually impressed upon her how bright and how talented she was, and that she could not settle for a "B"! Her old friends, the encyclopedia volumes, were her constant companions. "Look it up! Look it up!" her dad would say. And it wasn't enough that she learn just what she had to for school; Dad was fascinated by all kinds of things. He read every night and shared his books, papers, and the conversations about current events that he had with customers at the shop. The family sat around the dinner table, discussing current events, the presidential election, or the worrisome spread of communism. You couldn't be a passive listener in this family. Dad would say, "What do you think, Judy?" and it wasn't enough to say, "I didn't understand what you were talking about." Dad would then say, "What didn't you understand?" or "Which part of that were you not sure of?" or "Look it up, look it up!" They all laughed at Dad's fervor, and his way of sweeping everybody up in it. Judy was aware that other families weren't quite like hers, but she was proud of her dad. He was smart — really smart — and everybody loved him. He knew everybody in the neighborhood, and when he went out to walk the dogs, it would sometimes take an hour or more, because he'd have to stop several times to run down the state of the world with the neighbors. Ilse would smile affectionately and shake her head. Her brother's friends and all the relatives were always at their house, and more often than not, there was someone other than just their family at the dinner table.

Ilse, for her part, quietly urged her daughter on. She was less intense with instilling in Judy her own expectations that she should do well, but nevertheless, the message came through loud and clear. Judy had begun voice lessons, and she knew her mother was impressed with her skill on the piano. Ilse would always question Judy about school. She knew that her mom had frequent meetings with the teachers at school, and Ilse's message was always the same — you must give her the same opportunity to learn as the other kids have. You must acknowledge that she's bright and capable, and teach her what she needs to know. You cannot settle for less. Every issue was a variation on that same theme — over and over again.

It wasn't just at home; Judy had begun to attend Camp Oakhurst with other handicapped kids. She had expected the same kind of stuff she got from the teachers at school, but it didn't turn out that way. The "special" that came with being handicapped seemed to take on a different meaning there. It didn't seem to mean that you were less than, or better than, anyone else, but just that you all had this one thing in common. There was a strong sense that this "thing" that bound them together was a good thing. They all shared an understanding of themselves as being "different," but their differentness was okay. Well, maybe it was even better than okay. It was good when you had a handicap to not have to think about it too much — at camp, everybody else had one too, so it was fine! It was a revelation to Judy. She began to see that there were lots of different ways of looking at being handicapped, and that the trick was to figure out how to navigate your way through.

Ilse's shoulders sagged. She was tired and discouraged. Although she had managed to get her daughter into elementary school, she discovered that the city traditionally reverted to home instruction for handicapped children when they reached high school. The school board used the same rationale as before to deny her daughter the right to attend high school; the same ridiculous reasons as to why it simply could not be done. Ilse had seen that attending school was good for Judy. It might not have been the ideal educational experience, but the interaction with her peers had been good for her social development. Judy had many friends, and was comfortable with all kinds of people. The isolation that came with home instruction was not something she wanted her daughter to return to. When her arguments fell on deaf ears, she sought support from the March of Dimes. For many years, she had done volunteer work for the March of Dimes and felt they might be willing to take up her cause. They sympathized with her, but explained that the March of Dimes did not get involved with political issues. Ilse was bitterly disappointed; what issue could possibly be more important than education to parents of children with disabilities? It seemed that everybody wanted to prevent children from acquiring disabilities, but nobody wanted to deal with the very real, very practical issues faced by people with disabilities and their families. No one seemed to care, except the families themselves. Ilse thought about the other mothers who had supported her in her efforts to get Judy into school. By now, she knew many more parents of children with disabilities — Judy's classmates' parents. Ilse went home and made calls. She put together a group of parents and they began lobbying the school board for a policy change. They were relentless in the pressure they applied, until the school board finally backed down. In 1961, Judy finally entered high school.

High school was different, different than anything had been before. She was still bused out of district — this time to Sheepshead Bay High in East Flatbush. She still had homeroom with the handicapped students, but her classes were with non-disabled students. This was good and bad;

you were definitely considered "different," and this differentness wasn't considered a very good thing. Still, the work was more challenging, and after an initial, somewhat awkward time with the other kids, they seemed to accept her. Outside of the classroom, though, Judy found herself to be an "outsider." She couldn't participate in many after school activities because of the difficulty in getting home from school. Home was even busier than before; Ricky was off at college in Arizona, and Judy missed him a lot. Arizona might as well have been at the end of the world. Joey was working part-time at the butcher shop, and both of them were involved in a million activities: Boy Scouts, piano lessons, and voice lessons. As usual, Dad worked, read, and held court at the dinner table. However, the topics had altered somewhat. Now, instead of McCarthy, he was fascinated with the civil rights movement and the demonstrations against the war. A loyal Marine, he had difficulty with the disrespect the kids showed for their country but believed in their message of the importance of social equality and social conscience. Mom worked part time at Dad's shop, was president of the sisterhood at the synagogue, and head of the PTA. She still actively dogged the high school to make sure Judy got the best education Ilse could manage, and lent support to other parents with similar concerns. Mom and Dad often argued politics in front of them; in fact, they urged them to join in the arguments. Mom was a registered Republican and Dad was a fervent Democrat; although they often agreed, since Mom was a fairly liberal Republican, they sometimes did not. Judy was continually challenged to think through every side of an issue, and not to hesitate to join in the fray. Dad frequently shared his opinion that every American had a responsibility to inform him/herself and to take political action. It was what a democracy was all about, right? Now that the kids were older, Dad included them in outings to the theater, to concerts, and to art museums. "Culture is critical," he said, "it's what makes humans truly special. If you want to understand people, the beauty in people, learn their art and their culture."

Judy thrived in this environment. She was interested in boys, but did not date much. At school, most of the boys in her classes did not have disabilities, and were not particularly interested in dating someone who did. Camp was a different matter, though. At camp, the disability was not much of an issue, and she dated a couple of different boys. As she approached her senior year, she began to think ahead to her life after high school: what would she do? It was a foregone conclusion that she would follow her brother to college, but which college, to study what? Her one obvious talent was music. She loved music and was good at it, but was that what she wanted to do with her life? She had auditioned at Juilliard several months before, and although they had been encouraging, they said she was too young, and sent her home. She could re-audition, but her parents were concerned. Judy needed to do something that would allow her to support herself; although they were proud of their daughter's musical talent, they knew it was tough to make money at music. "What next?" Judy wondered. "What should I do?"

College and expanding horizons

Judy tore open the envelope — Okay! She was in! She would be going to Long Island University right here in Brooklyn. At least that was settled. Unfortunately, she would be majoring in speech and theater — it was not her first choice, but it was what the state rehabilitation agency would pay for. She had wanted to major in education, but her vocational rehabilitation counselor explained that they would pay for education only if students could demonstrate that they could get jobs related to their majors. The counselor patiently explained that no one would hire a girl in a wheelchair to teach in the public school system. With this major, however, Judy could get a job as a speech therapist. The problem was, she wanted to teach; she thought she would be good at it and did not see why she could not do it, but the counselor was adamant. "So, okay," thought Judy, "we'll play it her way." But in her head, Judy thought, "I'll bide my time a little. Something may yet come along to turn things my way."

The campus was a challenge. Bathrooms were difficult to manage and very often were completely inaccessible. She encountered difficulties with steps, narrow doorways, and occasional narrow minds. Using all the old, tired rationales, school officials refused her request for a dorm room but Judy persisted and finally persuaded them to relent. College was great in other ways, though; classmates were generally happy to help out when necessary, and the schoolwork was not difficult. There was a fair number of other students with disabilities, and they were able to share war stories and solutions to the practical problems of functioning in a university system that had never considered their needs. Judy also enjoyed the atmosphere of the university; she enjoyed the debate and the spirit of university life. People cared fervently about issues such as civil rights, poverty, and the Vietnam war. The students believed that if something was right, and you banded together to demand that people do the right thing, it could, and would, happen. The establishment, which was hell-bent on holding back new ideas and new ways of behaving, was under attack. Judy began to question why the establishment could also hold her back. There was nothing fair about not being able to get into the buildings that held the classes she wanted to take. She questioned the validity of policies that denied her the major and, thus, the career of her choice, simply because she used a wheelchair. As she listened to the debate about the plight of black people, she found herself identifying with them. She understood what it felt like to be treated differently and to have her choices restricted, while all the time knowing she was as capable as anyone. College taught her that there were people who would support individuals who took on the system. She learned about the NAACP and the ACLU. She quietly inquired about what it would take to get her teaching certificate. She was surprised and pleased to find that because there was a shortage of teachers, only twelve credits were needed. Without a word to anyone about what she was doing, she enrolled in an education course. On the first day of class, she waited for the teacher to single her out and demand an explanation for why she was attending a class where she didn't belong, but nothing happened. Nobody said a word; not her professors, not her advisor, not her rehabilitation counselor. Judy realized, however, that it probably wasn't because anything had changed. Rather, they probably just hadn't noticed. "Well," she thought, "let's see how far I can take this," and she registered for more education credits. Again, no one seemed to notice or to care, but Judy was worried. She had never heard of anyone who used a wheelchair being hired as a teacher. Judy picked up the phone and called the American Civil Liberties Union. They listened to her story, and advised her to continue on her current path of taking her education credits, and to call them if she had a problem. She never did have a problem; Judy graduated in 1970, ready to take the New York State teaching exam.

Taking a stand

She had a problem. A big problem. A really, really, really, big problem. Judy had passed the written exam with flying colors. She had passed the oral exam with flying colors. She had flunked the medical exam cold: polio. Wheelchair. Unfit. Period.

Judy was crushed, she was frustrated, and she was angry. She commiserated with her family and friends who, to a person, felt that she was being treated unfairly. Her mom and dad tried to help her sort it out, making suggestions and offering support. How could they have denied her? Hadn't she proven her fitness by graduating with every requirement met, and passing the exam? Her friends shared her anger. One of Judy's friends was a student reporter for the *New York Times*. He was really interested, and asked lots of questions. He asked Judy, "If I can get someone to write a story about you, will you agree to it?" Judy did not hesitate for even a minute. "Absolutely!" she replied. Several days later, a reporter from the *Times* called her. She again went over the story and shared her feelings about why this was wrong. Not wrong simply because it would prevent her, Judy Heumann, from teaching, but because policies like these prevented all people with disabilities from access to the same rights others enjoyed without question. This was a simple case of discrimination, and the only basis for their discrimination was her handicap, her use of a wheelchair. It was wrong.

The next day, Judy held her breath as she read the headline over the editorial "*You Can Be President, Not Teacher, with Polio.*" It was passionate, it was to the point, and it was all about her. The day was a blur of phone calls, and Judy was amazed. It seemed there was a lot of interest not only from family and friends, but she was getting calls from strangers. Then came a truly amazing call: NBC's *Today Show* wanted to interview her. Bob Herman, who seemed sympathetic to her situation, interviewed Judy. Then came more calls, this time from all over the country, and lots of letters with suggestions, offers of help, and general "Go get 'em, girl!" sentiments.

Judy sifted through all the information and weighed her next step. There was a strong tide of sentiment in her favor, but she knew that the board of education would be a formidable opponent. She had already taken all of the polite routes; it would now mean playing hardball. She knew if she took the next step, she was entering into new territory, but what else could she do? She was right, she knew she was right, and she wasn't going to back down. Judy searched for the business card she had tucked away a few days earlier, for a law firm that specialized in civil law. She squared her shoulders, set her jaw, and picked up the phone. "Here goes," she said aloud, and started dialing the number.

When it became apparent that they would lose the case, the board of education settled out of court. Judy started teaching that September at the same elementary school she had attended as a child. The fanfare that had accompanied her legal action quieted, but something had been awakened in Judy that she hadn't known was there. Just because she had gotten her teaching job did not mean that there were not millions of people with disabilities out there suffering the same abuses she had. She had friends who had similar problems, and Judy knew that just because she had been successful in opening one door, many others remained closed to her. The experience with her teaching certificate had taught Judy not to expect anything unless she fought and scraped for it, and she knew there was strength in numbers. The more Judy discussed these issues with her friends, the more they became convinced that they needed to do something about it. They weren't exactly sure what they needed to do, but the more she talked with others, the stronger and more determined she felt that together, they would be able to have an impact on the problems. Judy and her friends decided to respond to all the letters and phone calls she had received, to see whether any of those people would want to get together to discuss the situation. They set up a meeting and started making phone calls. The commonalities among the people were astounding; they were all dealing with the same barriers and individually feeling frustrated by their inability to do anything about it. Over time, the meetings grew in size. The group began to get organized around various subjects, and in February came up with a name for themselves: Disabled in Action, or DIA.

The following September, Judy began her new job. She loved teaching. She knew she was good at it, and felt she was adding something important to the children's lives. The school was still a regular school with special-ed classes located in a separate wing. After she had been there for almost a year, the principal approached her and said, "Judy, how would you feel about teaching the regular second grade class?" Judy had mixed feelings about it. She felt that one of the most important things she provided to her students was being a role model — a real, live, disabled grown-up who was doing exactly what she wanted to do. On the other hand, she realized that this would be ground-breaking. If she were given the chance to teach in a regular classroom, none of those students would ever again be able to look at a person with a disability as a poor unfortunate person who couldn't do anything for him or herself. This was another barrier that needed to be broken. They discussed it and decided to move the second grade class from the second floor to the first floor, and so, in her second year of teaching, Judy taught nondisabled students.

Throughout this period, Judy was actively involved in DIA, and helped orchestrate efforts to obtain curb cuts, and to advocate for ramps and physical accessibility. Members of the group grew more and more active, and honed their advocacy skills. The more work they took on, the more work there was to do. The group demonstrated against the Jerry Lewis telethon with its "Give to the poor, pitiful, handicapped children" theme. They worked hard to shut down the sheltered workshops, and to promote de-institutionalization. They continued to use "in-your-face" tactics, including demonstrations and protests, whenever polite inquiries were ignored, which was just about always. Judy was shocked at some of the things she discovered. One of the lowest hours of her life occurred when she confronted the truth about the abuses suffered by individuals with disabilities at a "treatment" facility called Willowbrook, and one of her greatest triumphs was the role DIA played in helping to close it down. Willowbrook was a large institution on Long Island which treated mentally disabled individuals. When a newspaper article revealed the atrocities occurring within the institution, DIA joined in the general outcry. In time, Judy decided to go and see the place for herself. She and another woman, who did not have a disability, went to Willowbrook and asked to see the facility. Judy was told that although they would allow the woman accompanying her to go inside, she could not enter because she was in a wheelchair and might hurt herself. Judy protested, so they asked her to sign a release form. When she refused, they flatly denied her entry to the facility. Judy was angry. What irony; the facility had freely abused its residents for years, and were now concerned that she might hurt herself. What garbage! DIA continued with its community activism. They developed valuable contacts in the community, and found a few key allies in government. The group became political, and advocated strongly for many pieces of legislation that had the potential to affect the lives, for the better, of people with disabilities. Members of DIA participated in the Washington, D.C. demonstration at the Lincoln Memorial when President Nixon vetoed a spending bill designed to fund disability programs. With a group of disabled Vietnam war vets, Judy took part in a takeover of Nixon's New York re-election headquarters to demand a public debate with President Nixon.

As she continued her work, Judy found that her political activism was taking over more and more of her life. She found that she was really very good at advocacy; she shared the passion of the activists, but also recognized the power of words. Her participation in the kitchen debates of her youth served her well, as she argued her points with precision and power. Lessons learned from her mother taught her to be persistent and not to back down. Judy was coming to the attention of policymakers and politicians who were sympathetic to her struggle.

Teaching continued to be important, but more and more, Judy began to feel that she might perhaps make her biggest contribution through advocacy, rather than education. She decided to return to grad school and went to Berkeley. At the end of her first year of grad school, Judy had to do an eighteen-month placement. She lucked out. While she was in New York, she had met Senator Harrison Williams through DIA. A friend called to tell her there was an opening for a legislative assistant in Senator Williams' office. At that time, Senator Williams was the chair of the Labor and Public Welfare Committee. Judy landed the job, and was suddenly in the thick of things. She learned how the political system worked (and sometimes didn't work). Her role was to act as a bridge between the people whose lives were being affected by the various legislative actions taken up by the committee, and the politicians actually crafting and passing the laws. In this capacity, she had the opportunity to work on two pieces of legislation that had great personal meaning to her: Public Law 94-142, and Section 504 of the Rehabilitation Act.

Public Law 94-142 was called the Education of All Handicapped Children Act, and for children with disabilities, it held the promise of correcting many of the inequities of the public school system. Children with disabilities would be guaranteed an equal and, whenever possible, integrated, educational experience. For the first time, the public school system would be required to accommodate the disabilities of children and to offer them a quality educational experience tailored to their individual needs.

Judy also worked on changes to the Rehabilitation Act which would guarantee basic civil rights, in terms of access and non-discrimination, to buildings and programs funded with federal dollars. When the Rehabilitation Act of 1973 passed with an entire title (Title V) dedicated to the civil rights of individuals with disabilities, Judy celebrated a small personal triumph. Other parts of the same act required the state rehabilitation agencies to actively involve disabled vocational rehabilitation clients in decisions about their own career goals and rehabilitation plans.

The Berkeley years

In 1975, Judy went to California at the invitation of Ed Roberts, the founder of the Berkeley Center for Independent Living. The center had grown out of a need for students at Berkeley to band together and advocate for accessibility on their campus, but had begun to move in the direction of doing many of the same things as DIA. California was a revelation: the state VR agency provided services not offered by the agency in New York, such as personal care attendants and van lifts. Perhaps more importantly, Judy found disabled people who had banded together and who shared a common identity. The energy in California was electric, and there was much support in the Berkeley environment for the kind of political activism that Judy had come to believe was absolutely necessary. Judy became the deputy director of the CIL. At that time, the CIL primarily assisted adults with physical disabilities. Judy, however, was painfully aware that there were many other disability groups that needed assistance and representation. She worked to expand the CIL's purview to children with disabilities and to those with cognitive, psychiatric, and substance-abuse disabilities. Since it was apparent that the need for employment was not being sufficiently met by the state vocational rehabilitation agency, she also worked to strengthen the employment program. The CIL was eventually able to have a huge impact on employment, when Ed Roberts was appointed commissioner for the California Vocational Rehabilitation Agency. A strong believer in the CIL's ability to effect change, Roberts was determined to get CILs established across California. Judy helped the legislators understand what CILs were all about, and her knowledge of the Washington political scene was instrumental in influencing the passage of federal independent-living legislation. Her testimony at a public hearing added to the powerful voices of other concerned individuals: a disabled child, a teacher, employers — all concerned with providing a mechanism for ensuring that people with disabilities would have a means of supporting each other, in accessing the rights afforded to others. While the federal CIL legislation eventually passed in 1978, there would be other, more difficult, battles ahead.

Roberts and Heumann found themselves at the center of a political blockade to stop implementation of legislation critical to the civil rights of individuals with disabilities. Section 504 of the 1973 Rehabilitation Act, had slipped past legislators largely unnoticed, but when the U.S. Department of Health, Education and Welfare began to weigh the practical implications of implementing the legislation, they estimated that it would cost millions of dollars. The Ford administration dealt with the problem by stalling it, and the draft regulations that would implement the law remained unissued. Jimmy Carter seized upon the issue in his presidential campaign, and promised to complete the regulations. The job fell to Carter's secretary of HEW, Joseph Califano. Upon initial review, Califano, too, became alarmed, and undertook an effort to rewrite the regulations. Delay followed delay, amid rumors that the proposed changes to the draft regulations would significantly lessen the protections currently provided. Implementation of the Education of All Handicapped Children Act had also been delayed for similar reasons since its passage in 1975, and HEW seemed unwilling to move forward. Califano refused to act, even when a disability organization called the American Coalition of Citizens with Disabilities (ACCD), headed by Frank Bowe, demanded at a candlelight vigil outside of Califano's home, that he release the regulations immediately. Bowe's group contacted other disability groups across the nation, and three days later, disability activists staged demonstrations in Washington, D.C. and HEW's eight regional offices. The Washington, D.C. demonstration caved in within twenty-eight hours when Califano, in his anger and indignation at the protesters, refused to allow food, or any form of communication, to flow in or out. One by one, the protests broke up in response to the angry retaliation, until there remained one lone group of hold-outs: Judy Heumann's demonstrators occupied the sixth floor of the San Francisco regional HEW office for twenty-five days. Heumann was furious at the treatment the demonstrators had received in other cities, and she and her fellow demonstrators resolved to "hang tough." The demonstrators were deprived of food, necessary medical supplies, and hygiene articles. The plight of, and the courage of, the protestors caught the attention of the media, however, and the message flashed around the world, "These individuals are willing to put their lives on the line for a chance at equal treatment under the law." Their passion for their cause and their determination to triumph despite all odds only increased with the press coverage. They received support from unexpected places, including a state representative who insisted, about a week into the demonstration, that food for the demonstrators be allowed in. The mayor of San Francisco provided air mattresses, and hoses with shower heads. Local stores, restaurants, and civil rights groups donated food and supplies. Sympathetic building employees smuggled food and information back and forth from the building. Califano, in desperation, attempted to bargain with the demonstrators, offering to pass a modified version, one that the demonstrators found completely unacceptable. Judy railed at the suggestion that the law allow for segregated schools for children with disabilities, and pronounced the changes abominable. She decried the attempts at enforced segregation, blatantly stating that they would not accept it. She forcefully stated that the demonstrations and sit-ins would not stop until government understood that segregation of people with disabilities could not now, and would never again, be tolerated.

Finally, Califano gave in to the demonstrators, and to the mounting public sympathy for their cause, and signed the regulations with no changes, as well as the regulations for the Education of All Handicapped Children Act. The demonstrators left the building in triumph, with the knowledge that they had, together, achieved a great victory in the battle for the protection of their basic rights, and with a new sense of their own power to effect change.

But Judy knew that the battle was far from over. She was convinced that the answer to effective activism was in bringing together people with all kinds of disabilities, who had the will and the skills to fight for what they needed, and to develop and support their activism through communication, development of data to support their positions, and information-sharing. Unfortunately, the political climate was changing. In 1980, Ronald Reagan became president and began implementation of what Judy termed his "slash-and-burn" agenda. He and his administration were determined to decentralize and reduce the size of the federal government, with little regard, Judy felt, for the people who, in the process, were experiencing upheaval in their lives. Judy was fired from two different commissions under the Reagan administration, a feat she later would consider a point of pride. Reagan did, however, appoint Justin Dart to begin working on the ADA — a move that would have a significant impact later on.

Judy worked briefly with Ed Roberts at the California Department of Education, but this job was a political appointment, and after Jerry Brown stepped down as governor, they lost the appointments. Judy and Ed were aware that their days were numbered in their jobs, and as the term was ending, they talked about what they wanted to do.

In 1983, Judy co-founded the World Institute on Disability (WID) with Ed Roberts and Joan Leon. The World Institute on Disability was a public-policy, research, and training organization based in Oakland, California. The WID worked on a number of issues, including research to support the establishment of personal-assistant services, research suggesting a need to focus on the issues of aging and disability, and others. The WID also developed a focus on international work. Judy had visited the wheelchair Paralympics in 1972, and had been amazed at the lack of poverty and the progressive social welfare policies. She was convinced that the U.S. could learn much from how other countries handled social and disability issues, and a primary mission of the WID was to foster international learning and sharing.

The culminating achievement of WID, however, may have been the role it played in the development and passage of the Americans with Disabilities Act (ADA). Judy, Ed, and Joan joined together with numerous others, including Justin Dart, Patrisha Wright, and Evan Kemp to draft, and then push the 1990 Americans with Disabilities Act through Congress. The group was supported in its efforts by several legislators, including Senator Tom Harkin and his aide, Bobbie Silverstein. To support the legislation with one large voice, WID and Judy played a major role in bringing together coalitions of different disability groups. Judy testified before the joint committee about the kinds of discrimination that had occurred in her life and how she had felt. They encountered numerous obstacles, delays, and frustrations, but finally, on July 26, 1990, President Bush signed the legislation. It was a day of rejoicing for all those who had shared their vision of a society that would not exclude individuals with disabilities from full and equal participation in all spheres of life. Judy, like the others, knew that the Act would not mean instant equality, but she knew that this was a truly historic moment, and she knew the role she had played in making it come to pass. It was more than a little shocking when she stopped to consider that she, little Judy from Brooklyn, the fire hazard who had scared the school administrators to death, called a good number of people on Capitol Hill by their first names!

The Office of Special Education and Rehabilitative Services

Unfortunately, Judy was right about the fact that Public Law 94-142, now renamed "The Individuals with Disabilities Education Act" (IDEA) and the ADA would not mean instant equality. Judy was kept busy fending off assaults on the legislation and trying to encourage the government to support the regulatory bodies' efforts to ensure compliance. She was encouraged by the emerging candidacy of Governor Bill Clinton. She viewed him as a progressive leader who seemed to have a feel for the problems faced by ordinary people. She went to work on his campaign, and in December 1992, she received a call from Bobby Simpson, the chair of the President's Committee on People with Disabilities, asking what kind of role she might be interested in within the new administration. Judy thought long and hard; she knew any job she would be interested in would have to affect the lives of kids through seniors. It would have to allow for policy work with both people with, and without, disabilities. She would also need to be able to effect change within other federal agencies not focused on disabilities.

After careful consideration, and after an extensive FBI check, Judy was nominated and confirmed as President Clinton's appointee to the role of assistant secretary of the Office of Special Education and Rehabilitative Services (OSERS) at the U.S. Department of Education. Judy accepted the appointment and went to work administrating the government office which controlled the regulatory body for the state vocational rehabilitation programs; the Education for All Handicapped Children Act, which had been renamed the Individuals with Disabilities Education Act (IDEA); and the National Institute on Disability Rehabilitation and Research (NIDRR), a body which awards millions of dollars to research funds in the areas of disability and rehabilitation. Today, Judy's office writes the regulations that she fought so hard to pry loose from DHEW Secretary Califano almost two decades earlier. She interacts with lawmakers and regulators at the highest levels of government, and finds that she must still play the role of activist. There are still constant assaults on key disability civil rights legislation, and still much to do to make the laws and regs better, and more responsive, to the changing needs of people with disabilities. One of the greatest challenges in her role as assistant secretary has been the reauthorization of the IDEA. Judy has given speeches, has published papers, and has campaigned tirelessly to ensure the reauthorization of the legislation, and to ensure that the provisions of the IDEA remain intact. At the signing ceremony, on June 4, 1997, Judy addressed the assembled officials and guests, and eloquently stated the significance of the accomplishments of her office, and of all of the individuals who had helped to bring the reauthorization of the IDEA to fruition:

> Today we can see a future where we finally put an end to the divisive, false argument that goes "something for your child means something less for my child." If the American experience tells us anything, it is that expanding opportunity lifts us all up. Let us be a proud nation that takes responsibility for all our children... We have come a long way, but we know that we can and must do better. Making progress will require continued partnership, aggressive collaboration, and a love for all children. This Act will give disabled young people more opportunities for quality education and meaningful employment than ever before in our nation's history. This is a splendid day of reaffirmation and promise...Now the real work begins.

Looking back on her work as assistant secretary, Judy smiles at comparisons between what she thought the work would be and what it has turned out to be. She has found the volume of work and the diversity of issues that she has to address to be beyond what she, or maybe anyone, could possibly have imagined. But the job has provided a platform from which many of her goals have been able to be met. She has been able to affect governmental programs in positive ways. She has encouraged the Department of Education to focus on disability issues outside and apart from OSERS. Her office staff members now serve on committees within other offices. She has worked, with considerable success, to create an office where different constituencies feel welcome, and where disability groups can take a role that is much more "hands-on" and be more actively involved. She believes parents have become more involved in school reform, and welcomes their participation. Conversely, she has been able to form coalitions with others in the administration on issues separate from, yet important to, people with disabilities. For example, Judy was actively involved in the development of the First U.S. International Women's Conference.

Judy counts the passage of the IDEA as a major victory for her office. The legislation came out of her office, and they won many significant battles to get the legislation passed, with numerous qualitative changes which have the potential to significantly improve the education of children with disabilities. She knows, however, that the battles are far from over. Now, her office must draft the regulations to implement the legislation, and enforcement of the regulations will be a huge challenge. She also knows that there is much work still to be completed on the Workforce Investment Act.

Although there is much left to do, Judy knows that there will be another administration change, and that she will once again have to think about what she wants to do. She really doesn't know, and it worries her some. On the other hand, she knows that opportunities have a way of emerging when you least expect them. She has faith that, once again, opportunity will probably come looking for her, as it always has.

****

It's been a long day. And it's not over. She checks her watch: it's 4:40 P.M. She has twenty minutes to get over to the reception for the National Rehab Association Governmental Affairs group, and then, finally, she and her husband will have a few minutes to themselves before bedtime. Judy's eyes scan her desk, surveying it for unresolved issues and loose ends. Is there anything left that can't wait until tomorrow? Her eyes alight upon the pink phone message from her mother — "Urgent!" She thinks back to the morning — her bout with the elevator — her fear of being late for the teleconference — the urgency in her mother's voice as she relayed the story of the new family from out of town, with the daughter who wants to study medicine. It *is* urgent to her mother, and it's urgent to her, too — for so many, many reasons. Judy smiles at the thought of her mother's indignation over the "system's" treatment of her friend's beautiful, smart daughter. She picks up the phone and calls home. "Hi Ma. How are you doing?...So what are their names?...uh, huh...their phone number?"

Sara pauses outside Judy's door. She wants to give Judy a couple of messages before she leaves the office for the day, but when she hears the conversation, she smiles to herself. She knows Judy is tired, knows her day is not over yet, but she also knows Judy is doing what she loves best. She flips out the light in the outer office, sticks the messages on the door, cracks open the door and catches Judy's eye. She points to the messages, and waves at Judy. Judy waves back, and continues her discussion. As Sara leaves the office, she thinks back to a speech Judy once made, where she relayed her mother's tireless efforts to get her into school. Referring to her mother, Judy had said "She is one of the toughest kinds of women you'll ever met — a housewife from Brooklyn, New York!"

"Different packaging, but the same stuff," Sara thinks to herself, closing the door on the circle of light pooling around the door.

chapter five

Frank Bowe

Brian T. McMahon

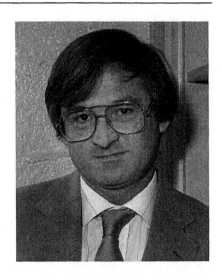

The discovery

Frank Bowe's story begins in that very-different country that was America in the late 1930s. In 1937, Lewisburg, Pennsylvania was nearly a two-hour drive north of Harrisburg on the Susquehanna River. It was a quiet town of 5000 people, most of whom were involved with either the Federal Penitentiary or Bucknell University. This is where nineteen-year-old Francis G. Bowe of New York City accepted a manufacturing job from a friend in neighboring Milton. This is where, in 1941, he met Kitty Windsor, the daughter of a local attorney. The two married in 1943, before Francis shipped out to France and Germany to serve in the Army. Their son, Frank was born in 1947, his sister Robin in 1949.

Beginning at the age of one, Frank contracted measles on two, and possibly three, occasions. He was unable to develop an immunity to the disease. To manage a frighteningly high fever, the doctor prescribed a new "miracle drug," injectable streptomycin. Shortly thereafter, his parents noticed that Frank was becoming progressively quieter and withdrawn. Suspecting the worst, Dad devised his own test of the young boy's hearing. First, he would attempt to awaken young Frank in the early morning, using loud words and noises. He thought perhaps he was a deep sleeper. But soon, Frank no longer noticed the sounds of boats on the river or the sound

1-57444-083-7/00/$0.00+$.50
© 2000 by CRC Press LLC

of the car bringing Dad home for lunch. Dad, banging books, crept up on
Frank when he was playing with building blocks. There was no response
to the banging.

After extensive testing at the Geisinger Medical Center, doctors finally
confirmed that Frank's profound hearing impairment was permanent. The
family was referred to Dr. Edmund J. Fowler, Jr. at Columbia-Presbyterian
Medical Center in Manhattan. Dr. Fowler proceeded with days of tests and
research. He concluded that Frank was likely born a hearing child, but lost
his hearing in his second year, due to recurrent measles, the streptomycin,
or a combination thereof. He was intrigued by Frank, because, due to his
parents' vigilance, he was a subject whose hearing loss was of recent onset,
and thus, his speech was better than that of congenitally deaf children. He
wanted to perform further tests to establish the etiology, but Frank was tired
of being poked and prodded. His mother took him home.

Frank Bowe summarizes in these words the experience of growing up deaf:

> Deafness means being alone.
> You don't hear the sounds people make as they move
> about in the house; there is no connection with others
> unless you can see them.
> Being deaf, too, means that even when others are in
> the room with you, you don't know what they say to
> each other.
> There is no incidental learning. None.
> Your sister learns by overhearing conversations be-
> tween your parents. She learns by listening to the radio
> while she plays with her toys. She learns by watching
> television programs.
> She learns by talking to her friends.
> You do none of this.
> You sit quietly, doing whatever you happen to be do-
> ing, oblivious to what is going on around you.
> It means, as well, that whenever a family member
> wants to tell or ask you something, that individual
> must attract your attention by touching you or moving
> within your field of vision.
> And then begins the slow, agonizing, emotionally
> draining process of communicating.
> Words are repeated until they are understood. Ideas
> are expressed, three, four, or five times through differ-
> ent words and different sentences. You catch a word
> here, a word there, and guess about the rest.
> Very quickly, despite their love for you and desire to
> include you in the daily life of the family, your parents
> and siblings talk to you only when necessary.
> There is no idle chitchat, no talking for relaxation.

> You do not pick up the bits and pieces of someone's
> character, personality, interests, and worries that others
> get in the course of talking "about nothing."
> You know your mother, your dad, and your sister only
> from what you see them do and say directly to you.
> Slowly, surely, your isolation grows. (*Changing the
> Rules*, 1986, p. 21)

Dad's way, the hard way

Mother taught Frank to read even before kindergarten. Long before the concepts of special education and "mainstreaming" became widespread, families such as the Bowes were faced with the choice of regular vs. "special" schools. Doctors and educators were unanimous in their advice to the family that Frank should go to a special school, but for Dad it was a closed subject. Dad was adamant that Frank should never be permitted to escape from anything just because it might be hard. Frank must confront head-on any problem he encountered, without slinking away or being excused on the grounds of his deafness. Although Frank later questioned the wisdom of this decision, there is no doubt that his persistence and tenacity resulted partly from Dad's influence.

In the beginning, Frank attended public schools, where amplification devices and speech reading lessons offered some relief from his social isolation, but signing was strictly prohibited. He enrolled in hundreds of hours of boring lip-reading classes, offered by a student teacher at neighboring Bloomsburg Teachers College. The classes made him anxious about his future in school and beyond. He came to realize that only 30% of a person's conversation appears legibly on the lips, so lip-reading was an imperfect business at best. Consequently, Frank sat in silent turmoil throughout many of his elementary, junior-high, and high-school years and then well into college.

One day, Frank checked out a *Boy Scout Handbook* from the library. He was not interested in scouting, but he was intensely interested in a page of small sketches showing how the letters of the alphabet, and some numbers, could be made by using hand signs. With these signs, deaf people (and Scouts) could learn to "talk with their hands." Excitedly, Frank shared his discovery with his parents. Dad immediately dismissed the idea:

> Frank, I knew this day was going to come...every doc-
> tor, everybody...they were so urgent in condemning
> signs...because if you learn to sign, you won't talk.
> You won't learn to lip-read. You'll only be able to talk
> with those few people who know that hand language.
> We didn't bring you up to toss you into a ghetto. Our
> choice was this: either we bring you up in a hearing
> world, which happens to be our world, or we give you

over to the deaf world. That means giving you up. You
mean too much to us to do that. Besides, the hard way
is the best way. (*Changing the Rules*, 1986, p. 92).

Scores of anecdotes about Frank Bowe's coming of age are candidly reported
in his 1986 autobiography, *Changing the Rules*. Some are specific to his deafness, others describe the normal, but sometimes humorous and awkward,
aspects of development: schooling, peer conflicts, friendships, Little League,
tennis, and dating. Regarding education, however, it is clear that there was
little of what we now term "accommodations" for Frank's hearing loss.
    Looking back, Frank Bowe says:

> I can smile about it now, but my growing-up years
> were painful. The world just didn't make sense to me.
> As an example: At five years of age, I worked really
> hard to prepare for kindergarten (isn't that an absur-
> dity in itself?), only to discover it was largely a matter
> of singing songs. That was one of my first signals that
> the world was not about to bend, even one inch, for
> me. The school never gave me an interpreter, a noteta-
> ker, a tutor, or any other kind of help, all the way
> throughout twelfth grade.
> In fact, in junior high school, I had to take two full
> years of music. To make matters worse, instead of
> handing out test sheets, the music teacher spoke each
> question out loud. Not understanding the questions —
> and not having understood some 90% of the lecture
> anyway — I was setting all-time records for ineptitude.
> I don't think anyone else in the history of the school
> had ever received an "F" in music! The final exam
> consisted solely of listening to a record and interpret-
> ing it.
> It was pointless, absurd. Many of us who are now
> adults had to put up with these kinds of things as
> children and youth. I'm glad today's young people
> with disabilities grow up in a more rational world.
> I guess you need to know a lot about deafness to un-
> derstand this, but learning to read the English lan-
> guage was hardest of all. It took me until I was in ninth
> grade before I could read well enough to learn any-
> thing else. I can tell you now — learning to read was
> the hardest thing I will ever have to do. That imbues
> me with a real confidence: I did *that*!
> Growing up deaf in that time and place, with no in-
> terpreters, no captions, no social life at all…being a
> stranger in a strange land for all those years…it is hard

> to imagine a childhood and adolescence more de-
> signed to isolate me.
> Looking back, it was oppressive. I think my sense of
> humor, which runs to the sardonic, comes from that.
> (Personal communication, 1997).

Despite average grades early on, Frank chose an academic "college preparatory" track in high school, rather than the "vocational" track prescribed
for other students with disabilities. Young Frank compensated for the limited
exchanges of information in the classroom by enthusiastically engaging in
an inordinate amount and variety of reading. One book in particular, Ayn
Rand's *The Fountainhead*, impressed upon him that great things were possible, even for him.

This notion was further bolstered by an intensive summer testing program at Bucknell University's counseling center, where renowned counselor
Allen Ivey confirmed that Frank had the aptitude and ability to compete at
a high academic level. Frank sought to excel in academics and, in 1965,
graduated thirteenth in a class of 188, a remarkable improvement from his
earlier years. He also excelled at tennis, and found himself in high demand
as a competitor and doubles partner. As he discovered areas in which he
excelled, Frank found that the social distance he experienced as a youth
began to dissipate somewhat.

Frank decided to go to Western Maryland College. He majored in
English, philosophy, and religion. As captain of the tennis team, and through
his fraternity membership, Frank made many friends. His involvement in a
men's leadership society, Omicron Delta Kappa, was also meaningful.
Frank's value system was deeply and permanently influenced by the social-
political events of the times. The assassinations of Martin Luther King, Jr.
and Robert F. Kennedy, the rising resistance to the accelerated U.S. involvement in Vietnam, the cultural revolution surrounding sex and drugs, and
the active civil rights movement were among the events that would affect
him for years. Civil rights became a subject of serious study for Frank. He
saw civil rights issues as the clear struggle between good and evil, and he
carefully analyzed the positions of the various stakeholders. Such analyses
provided the foundation for the strategies and tactics that would become
the tools of his advocacy work in the years ahead.

One day, as Frank was nearing graduation, an event occurred that would
forever change his life. While driving down a West Virginia highway, he
noticed that he was nearing Frederick, West Virginia, where there was a
school for the deaf.

> I might as well stop over at the school for the deaf, I
> thought.
> A few minutes later, I found myself escorted to a class-
> room filled with eleven- and twelve-year-olds. Drop-
> ping to one knee, I talked with each of them. They

flickered their fingers and swept their hands in rapid
gestures, none of which I understood. But they seemed
fascinated by my hearing aid.

One boy, whose name tag said he was Danny, walked
up to me, pointed to me, and then to himself. Then he
made a simple gesture joining the two of us.

"He's saying 'same,'" my escort translated.

I turned back to Danny.

"Same," I signed.

His face lit up. A few moments later, the group crowded around me. It was all my escort could do to keep
up with the questions. Where was I from? When had
I become deaf? What did I do? Did I have any brothers
or sisters?

I answered all the questions, then begged to depart. I
was overcome with emotion, just overwhelmed at a
sudden and very powerful sense of kinship, of belong-
ing, and, yes, of being needed. I knew I had little to
offer those kids, other than myself.

But I knew where to learn what I had to know:
Gallaudet. (*Changing the Rules*, 1986, p. 164).

Then and there, Frank vowed to do something to help the "little Franks,"
but he realized that good intentions were not enough. He would need to
acquire the ability to provide a good education to kids like these. In 1969,
Frank graduated *summa cum laude* from Western Maryland College. His
parents were proud of his intention to accept a fellowship at Gallaudet
College to pursue a master's degree in education of the deaf.

The Gallaudet College experience

Suddenly, Frank Bowe was immersed in deaf language and culture. In the
course of his studies, McCay Vernon, a scholar on the psychology of deafness,
helped to arrange for Frank a research assistantship with the federal Rehabilitation Services Administration (RSA). The assistantship provided exposure to state-of-the-art research on sensory impairments. It also enabled
Frank to establish a number of personal contacts in Washington, including
Mary Switzer, the legendary director of RSA.

It took Frank nearly a year to master sign language. His own experience
convinced him that sign language was in no way harmful to deaf children.
For the first time, Frank was able to understand what people were saying
to each other:

I could see it, right there in front of me.
I spent hour after hour sitting in group rooms, watching one conversation after another.

It was a wonderful, settling experience. At last, I knew.
This huge mystery I had wondered about for years.
On one level, I was disappointed: most of the conversations were incredibly dull. Yet on another level, I was
fascinated. What people actually say is only part of
what they mean. I could see two people who knew
each other well, interrupting each other, finishing the
other's sentences. I could see, too, a kind of verbal
shorthand between two close friends, a great deal left
unspoken. (*Changing the Rules*, 1986, p. 169).

During this same period, a virtual explosion was taking place in research on
the subject of deafness. By 1970, there was general consensus that "total
communication" (which includes speech, lip-reading, finger spelling, and
sign language) was the best communication strategy to adopt with deaf
children. Frank's parents had been wrong about sign language. Naturally,
he wanted to shared his discovery with his parents. Given the information
available to them at the time, Frank accepted that they had made the only
decision that made sense to them. When it was discussed, however, Dad
remained intransigent, defending his original position. Frank asked them to
learn some fingerspelling and a few signs, so that he could share within the
family all the nuances of communication he had discovered. But they
refused, and although Frank accepted this at an intellectual level, he was
deeply disappointed.

Learning from kids, scholars, and mentors

As graduation neared, Frank was tempted by the prospects of immediate
doctoral studies and an academic career. However, he remembered his commitment to the kids in central Pennsylvania, who were sorely in need of
special education services. Bloomsburg Teachers College provided him with
precisely the opportunity he sought. Frank was hired to locate children in
need, screen and select promising candidates, develop and teach the necessary classes, and manage all aspects of a program to enhance their education.
Frank assembled his first group of seven students — Glenda, Chris, Craig,
Pamela, Steve, Tina, and Hope — and the program flourished. He also taught
sign language to scores of student teachers and therapists, and enlisted each
one in service to the children. There were families to be counseled and
activities to be organized, but this was a labor of love. Frank demonstrated
the effectiveness of the program, and when the school district committed
the resources necessary for its expansion, he concluded that his work there
was done, and that it was time to move on.

In 1972, Frank enrolled in a rigorous Ph.D. program in educational
psychology at New York University, working full time as a researcher and
teaching classes in deafness education and rehabilitation. His research
resulted in scores of technical reports and scholarly presentations, given from

coast to coast. While he was at NYU, he met Phyllis Schwartz, and after a six-month courtship, the two were married, and settled into an apartment at Washington Square Village. The couple were soon blessed with two healthy daughters, Doran and Whitney.

As his doctoral studies approached a successful conclusion, Frank befriended Eunice Fiorito, a political in-fighter, and director of the New York City Mayor's Office for the Handicapped. Fiorito, a blind psychiatric social worker was an inspiration to Frank Bowe. In 1975, she founded the American Coalition of Citizens with Disabilities (ACCD). She described to Frank her dream of creating a national civil rights movement to be run by disabled people themselves, in order to achieve equal opportunity in every aspect of American life. She shared her conviction that it was the time for scores of *uni-disability* organizations to come together and accomplish *cross-disability* goals. After several meetings, Frank was convinced that ACCD was the appropriate vehicle to effect such changes, and that he and Eunice knew where to begin.

Section 504 of the 1973 Rehabilitation Act was now law. It was to become the prototype of the Americans with Disabilities Act, a so-called "bill of rights" for disabled Americans. In brief, Section 504 prohibited discrimination on the basis of physical or mental handicap in federally assisted programs:

> No otherwise qualified handicapped individual in the
> United States…shall, solely by reason of his handicap,
> be excluded from participation in, be denied the ben-
> efits of, or be subjected to discrimination under any
> program or activity receiving federal financial assis-
> tance (*Changing the Rules*, 1986, p. 183).

Due to the vast reach of U.S. government funds, these "programs and activities" included schools, colleges, state governments, hospitals, libraries, mass transit facilities, post offices, airports, and all others receiving or benefiting from federal grants. The language in Section 504 was so strong and so far-reaching that it had the potential to revolutionize the experience of living with a disability in America.

The law had been vetoed twice by President Nixon, due to presumed excessive costs. The first veto had really angered Frank Bowe, who was still a doctoral student. Cost had never been a consideration in the rights of other minorities. In the hope of encouraging a Congressional override, he joined with colleagues in Washington, D.C. to demonstrate. There, he met congressional staff members, including Lisa Walker, then working with Senator Harrison Williams, and Jack Duncan, who was with Representative John Brademas. This was the beginning of warm and lasting friendships that would serve Frank well in the years ahead. In dialogues with these colleagues, Frank Bowe's anger was tempered by the realization that the Democratic Congress was gearing up to challenge what was perceived as Nixon's imperial presidency. He came to view Congress as a "more-than-equal part-ner" with the executive branch, especially because of its power to override a presidential veto. "The president proposes, but Congress disposes" became more than a time-worn phrase. He would look to Congress for allies in the disability rights movement.

One of Frank Bowe's many early lessons was using his emotions to generate motivation and commitment, while balancing them with reason and diplomacy to achieve results. The second veto was subsequently over-ridden by the Senate, but three years after the 1976 enactment of the law, the U.S. Department of Health, Education, and Welfare (HEW) had yet to promulgate regulations for the enforcement of Section 504. In effect, this inaction "sidelined" Section 504 to the level of a platitude, a pronouncement, an empty promise which no one took seriously. The law had been enacted, but it was ineffective.

Never so alive

Frank and Eunice studied the problem, generating and evaluating various solutions. To realize the promise of 504, someone would have to put pressure on the executive branch of the federal government. Regulations would have to be completed and immediately approved. Eunice knew how to make this happen, and in May, she offered Frank Bowe the position of the chief exec-utive officer for ACCD. She candidly described the position as a 24-hour-per-day job of tilting at windmills — establishing, virtually from scratch, a headquarters office for a national organization, attracting the funds needed to operate that office, hiring staff, and battling the nation's top political officials for hotly controversial civil rights gains.

Frank hesitated; he was recently married and the young couple was expecting their first child in a few months. He had looked forward to a career as a researcher in learning and memory. Eunice Fiorito was asking for a five-year commitment of service, during which Frank could potentially improve the lives of millions of Americans. Learning and memory, she argued, would likely be more or less unchanged when he returned to his academic career. Frank Bowe relented; with the love and full support of Phyllis, he accepted the challenge.

Acting quickly, Frank established a presence for ACCD in the nation's capital. To be effective as a lobbyist, he needed information. He gathered all the necessary data, studied demographic statistics, judicial decisions, unpub-lished studies, sensitive memoranda, newspaper clippings, and the like, and scoured every source of information available to uncover, document, and detail the reality of discrimination against disabled Americans.

In January 1977, Joseph Califano was the incoming Secretary of HEW under President Jimmy Carter. Friendly but unfruitful meetings occurred with him. The issue of discrimination became a flash point for dozens of self-help organizations from coast to coast, and both funds and letters of support were forthcoming for ACCD.

More promises and requests for patience came from the secretary's office, but there was still no action. The Carter administration was concerned about costs and the extension of disability protection to persons with chemical dependency. Frank recognized that it was no longer a legal battle, but a political one. He travelled the country giving speeches to generate grass-roots support in local congressional districts. Frank determined that the solution to the problem was to put national pressure directly upon Joseph Califano. On March 18, 1977, Frank Bowe drafted a letter to the president, and sent a copy to Califano. The letter announced that, unless regulations were issued by April 4, three weeks hence, ACCD would mount a massive sit-down demonstration in every HEW regional office, from coast to coast. Jack Anderson ran the story in his syndicated column on March 26, headlined "Handicapped Plan 10-City Sit-in." Even members of Congress joined in the chorus of demands upon Califano.

What happened next came as a complete surprise to Frank Bowe: on April 4, Califano called a media press conference, and announced that he "endorsed" the demonstration, and required all HEW personnel to cooperate fully with the protesters in the exercise of their constitutionally protected free speech.

The demonstrations began, and in Washington, D.C., Califano himself received the group, promising to issue regulations "soon" and saying that they would be "fair." He said, "I thank the people here today for helping me draw the country's attention to the injustices this administration is deter-mined to end." And then, politely, he asked the demonstrators to leave.

During its first months in office, the worst of all nightmares ensued for the Carter administration. The demonstrators would not leave. They demanded, and received, donuts and coffee upon orders from Califano, and only withdrew from the D.C. offices when concerns mounted over the health of some of the protesters. The sit-in lasted even longer in several cities, including a full twenty-five days and nights in San Francisco. In some cities, protesters tried, but could not get arrested, due to inaccessible prisons. Disappointed at the pull-out at HEW headquarters, a California contingent, including Judy Heumann (see Chapter 4), flew to Washington. They picketed Califano's home, followed the Carters to church, and tried unsuccessfully to re-occupy HEW headquarters. Finally, all the protesters returned home, and the next day, April 28, 1977, Secretary Califano called a press conference to announce the promulgation of the regulations, which he had signed at 7:30 that morning. He said:

> The 504 regulations attack the discrimination, the de-
> meaning practices, and the injustices that have afflict-
> ed the nation's handicapped citizens. They reflect the
> recognition of Congress that most handicapped per-
> sons can lead proud and productive lives, despite their
> disabilities. They will usher in a new era of equality

> for handicapped individuals in which unfair barriers
> to self-sufficiency and decent treatment will begin to
> fall before the force of law. (*Changing the Rules*, 1986,
> p. 193).

The key aspects of Title V of the Rehabilitation Act of 1973 would now be implemented. Section 504's prohibition of discrimination on the basis of disability in any program or activity receiving or benefiting from federal financial assistance would have a profound, nationwide effect. Notably, it resulted in accessibility features at virtually every airport in the United States, as well as in most public schools, colleges, universities, libraries, hospitals, and social services agencies. Section 501 of Title V, which required federal agencies to practice nondiscrimination in employment, showed that people with disabilities could work effectively in a vast range of jobs, and that accommodating their limitations cost relatively little. However, no one involved in writing Section 501 could have anticipated the extent to which federal employment would plateau shortly after the requirements took effect, thus limiting Section 501's impact on reducing unemployment among Americans with disabilities.

Much the same scenario occurred with Section 502 of Title V, which required physical access to federal buildings, since relatively few had been erected in the years following enactment of the law. Section 503, which required affirmative action by private companies holding federal contracts (e.g., IBM had contracts to supply federal agencies with computers) had an effect much like that of Section 501: it showed that people with disabilities could be productive workers, and that accommodations could be inexpensive. However, most companies subject to Section 503 gradually "downsized" in the years after the requirement took effect.

Nonetheless, Title V of the Rehabilitation Act had the resounding effect of establishing vitally important precedents, showing that fair employment opportunities and barrier removal *could* occur in reasonable ways — and both were surprisingly affordable. In securing Congressional enactment of the Americans with Disabilities Act in 1990, both points were cited again and again. Title V also produced a body of case law which demonstrated that the definitions of such key terms as "qualified," "disability," and "reasonable accommodation," were viable and could be operationalized in the real world. This case law, the research results compiled by Frank Bowe and others, and the resurgence of coalition politics were the critical ingredients in the eventual passage of the most significant piece of civil rights legislation since 1964: the 1990 Americans with Disabilities Act (ADA).

With the HEW demonstrations in 1977, 30-year-old Frank Bowe emerged as an important spokesperson for the American disability rights movement. As ACCD's executive director, Frank was one of the first national leaders of this movement who was himself an individual with a disability. He used his exceptional research skills to study and document the public attitudes and government actions that precluded people with disabilities from equal participation

in American society; he also used his solid
presentation skills to articulate the cause of
disability rights in a manner, and at a level,
heretofore unprecedented. Frank realized
that success would depend largely upon his
ability to raise both money and consciousness regarding disability. For this, he would
turn to the power of the pen.

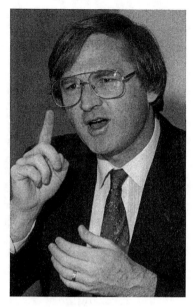

In his first book, *Handicapping America:
Barriers to Disabled People* (1978) Frank Bowe
identified six barriers to the full inclusion
of disabled citizens in American society:
architectural barriers, attitudinal barriers,
educational barriers, occupational barriers,
lack of legal recourse, and personal barriers.
He posited that *American society reinforced
these barriers* by persisting in the view that
persons with disabilities "cannot."

> For 200 years we have designed
> a nation for the average, able-bodied majority—we
> have created an image of disabled people that is per-
> haps the greatest barrier they face. America handicaps
> disabled people...and because that is true, we are
> handicapping America itself. (*Handicapping America*,
> 1978, p. *vii–viii*).

This was a radical view, which challenged the widely held belief that the
problem of disability was somehow within disabled persons themselves, and
it was their responsibility to adjust to society, not vice versa.

In 1980, Frank Bowe published his plan for achieving full inclusion of
people with disabilities. In *Rehabilitating America: Toward Independence for
Disabled and Elderly People*, Frank deliberately linked the status and future of
the disabled with elderly Americans. He appreciated the demographic reality
that disability and aging are correlated, and that the aging of America's baby
boomers would eventually give both disabled and elderly persons the enormous political muscle necessary to accomplish their goals. Once again, Frank
Bowe used his data and knowledge of research to argue forcefully that the
existing costs of a segregated America are far greater than the necessary
investment in accessibility, inclusion, mainstreaming, and rehabilitation.
Frank Bowe illustrated how such investments would eventually be recovered
through increased employment and a broadened tax base.

The book was received well, but with the usual rejoinder: "How can we
afford this?" Frank Bowe felt certain that resistance on economic grounds
was simply a disguise for the private discomfort felt by most Americans

regarding people with disabilities, and the age-old institutions and policies designed to "care" for them.

> We have created an image of disabled people that is perhaps the greatest barrier they face. We see the disability—the chrome and the leather, the guide dog, the hearing aid, the crutches—and look the other way. Just as we cannot seem to see the man in the policeman, so imposing are the uniform and the cultural expectations that go with it, so we cannot see the woman in the wheelchair. We do not see, nor do we look to find, her abilities, interests, and desires. (*Rehabilitating America*, 1980, p. *viii*).

During his tenure at ACCD from 1976 to 1981, Frank Bowe had many other notable achievements. In that period, he supervised a group of twenty, including attorneys, researchers, trainers, and administrative personnel. Under his leadership, ACCD achieved major legislative and regulatory gains in civil rights, transportation, Social Security, housing, education, rehabilitation, and assistive technology. He held several presidential appointments and advised the U.S. Congress Office of Technology Assessment. He consulted with the U.S. House of Representatives Committee on Science and Technology and drafted the original legislation that created both the National Institute of Disability and Rehabilitation Research (NIDRR) and the National Council on Disability (NCD). But most important, Frank presided over the coming together of the fragmented constituencies of the disability community to become a powerful force for progress. After completing his five-year commitment to Eunice Fiorito and the organization, Frank Bowe left ACCD in 1981. Due to divisions within the disability community, ACCD disbanded in 1986. Sadly, the country has been without a nationwide coalition dedicated to disability rights ever since.

Global concerns and the power of the pen

In 1979, while Frank was in the midst of his term as ACCD executive director, Secretary of State Cyrus Vance appointed Bowe as the head of the U.S. delegation to the United Nations' International Year of Disabled Persons. Prime Minister Menachem Begin invited him to Israel to make recommendations on programs for disabled war veterans and civilians. He also consulted with France, the United Kingdom, Japan, Canada, and the United Nations in Vienna and New York.

Bowe's international experience moved him to compile some stunning world-disability statistics. He observed that of 500 million disabled people worldwide, approximately 90% live in Third World countries. This realization sparked the beginning of a transformation in his approach:

> I have been struck repeatedly by the fact that one trag-
> ically wrong perception dominates the lives of the
> world's 500-million disabled citizens...that little, if
> anything, can be done to help these people; that they
> are more disabled than able; that they can't. As a result,
> the lives of these millions are unnecessarily deprived,
> difficult, and, often, short....at least three out of every
> five disabled individuals are not receiving even the
> most minimal kinds of education, rehabilitation, or
> other assistance they need to become independent,
> self-sufficient citizens....I lost most of what little faith
> I had in the power of mere words, statistics, and re-
> search reports. Rather, I came to believe, the abilities
> of disabled people had to be dramatized. People must
> be led to see and to believe that even the most severe
> and profound physical and mental disabilities are con-
> ditions that can be, have been, and are being overcome.
> (*Comeback*, 1981, p. 152).

Abraham Maslow, a famous psychologist from New York, was critical of
psychology as a study of mental illness. He felt that much more could be
learned by studying the "growing tip" of society, people he termed "self
actualized." Similarly, Bowe undertook an intensive investigation of the lives
of six people with varying disabilities whose lives seemed to exemplify the
simple but remarkable fact that disabled people *can*. Susan Daniels, Nansie
Sharpless, Eunice Fiorito, Stephen Hawking, Roger Meyers, and Robert
Smithdas were featured in Frank Bowe's 1981 book *Comeback: Six Remarkable
People Who Triumphed Over Disability*. Bowe found certain commonalities in
their development that led to his development of a "bill of rights" for the
disabled child:

- The right to be helped to become a fully developed person.
- The right to be granted as much freedom and independence as are
  other children of the family (the right to fail).
- The right to have one's abilities, not disabilities, treated as the critical
  factors for one's success.
- The right to have one's disability perceived as an obstacle to be overcome rather than as a crippling liability.
- The right to have unnecessary environmental barriers removed from
  the home.

He discovered that each of these successful individuals had parents who
understood without coddling, supported without overwhelming, and guided
without directing. He found that each person was disciplined, hard-working,

patient, curious, practical, friendly, and socially intelligent. Each sought information about disability, access to technology, quality education, and appropriate rehabilitation services. Finally, each had a realistic sense of self and a ribald sense of humor. In *Comeback*, Frank Bowe advocates for an international policy that will develop the support services that promote the development of these personal characteristics for disabled persons worldwide.

Frank Bowe was careful to consistently ground his arguments in economics and to defend his positions with facts and figures, not with personal anecdotes. At the urging of Russell Baxter, Arkansas director of vocational rehabilitation, and Vernon Glenn, director of the Arkansas Rehabilitation Research and Training Center, Frank Bowe accepted an appointment as a visiting professor at the University of Arkansas from 1981 to 1984. There he published a series of six books, including *Demographics and Disability: A Chartbook for Rehabilitation* (1983), *Disabled Adults in America* (1984), *Disabled Women in America* (1984), *The U.S. Census and Disabled Adults: The Fifty States and the District of Columbia* (1984), *Black Adults with Disabilities* (1985), and *Disabled Adults of Hispanic Origin* (1985). In these books, Frank Bowe accurately outlined, for the first time, the status of non-institutionalized, disabled Americans. Politicians and policymakers could no longer escape the facts:

- Approximately one in five adults is disabled.
- Over eight million disabled adults received no educational services.
- Five of six disabled persons were once non-disabled.
- More men than women are disabled.
- Most disabled people are unemployed or underemployed.
- In the South or in inner cities, most disabled people live below the poverty line.
- Disability is more prevalent among African-Americans.

Frank Bowe has authored or edited twenty-seven books, some of which have had significant international distribution, and more than seventy-five journal articles. Most of his writings concern the design and application of personal computers to help overcome barriers imposed by disability, public interest advocacy, the effects of social policy on disabled and elderly persons, and demographics of disability. Books he has authored include *Personal Computers and Special Needs; Birth to Five: Early Childhood Special Education; Access to Transportation; Coalition Building; Planning Effective Advocacy Programs;* and *I'm Deaf Too: Twelve Deaf Americans.* Edited works include *Participating Citizens; Self-help Groups in Rehabilitation;* and *Full Mobility.* Several of these works received awards from the President's Committee on Employment of People with Disabilities, the National Association for the Deaf, the American Library Association, and the National Conference of Christians and Jews. In 1981, Gallaudet College awarded Frank an honorary doctor of laws degree (L.L.D.).

Advocacy as a way of life

From 1984 to 1987, Frank Bowe served as director of research for the U.S. Architectural and Transportation Barriers Compliance Board. There he administered research contracts on building and telecommunications systems designed to benefit persons with disabilities, and senior citizens. From 1987 to 1989, Frank served as Region II RSA Commissioner (including New York, New Jersey, Puerto Rico, and the Virgin Islands) under Rehabilitation Services Administration (RSA) commissioner Justin Dart. There he administered $150 million in formula and discretionary grants. He supervised six state agencies for vocational rehabilitation and monitored hundreds of rehabilitation facilities, training programs, independent living centers, and other programs. During this period, Lois Beilin, then dean of the school of education at Hofstra University, approached Frank Bowe about a faculty position.

Frank Bowe's involvement with the Americans with Disabilities Act began in February 1988, when the first draft of the bill, written by Robert Burgdorf, a staff attorney for the National Council on Disability, was presented to the 100th Congress. Little happened that session, but 124 representatives and 26 senators signed on as co-sponsors. By the time the 101st Congress met in 1989, the bill had undergone significant revisions at the hand of Robert Silverstein. Frank Bowe's efforts would be primarily on the Senate side, working closely with Senate sponsors, such as Tom Harkin, Ted Kennedy, and David Durenberger. There were regular meetings, constant negotiations, and incessant faxes, proposing and revising specific legislative language. While considerable attention was drawn to the employment and public access provisions, Frank Bowe had particular interest in Title IV, which was reworked several times. Title IV required access to telecommunications for hearing- and speech-impaired persons who used Telecommunications Devices for the Deaf (TDDs). It would create a network of dual-party relay services in which operators translated text to voice, and *vice versa*, thus enabling all deaf and hearing persons to have unrestricted telephone conversations. In effect, it would give telephone access to between three and eleven million new customers. Title IV also called for the use of advanced technology in the future, as it becomes feasible. In today's terms, that means the use of speech-to-speech relay services, speech synthesizers, and video telephony. Frank Bowe himself uses an Intel Pentium MMX computer (optimized for video), which allows him to see the other caller and read signs or, with more difficulty, lips.

Once again, the itinerant Frank Bowe flew around the country giving speeches to encourage people to become active in shaping and supporting the legislation — people with sensory impairments, cognitive impairments, HIV infection, spinal-cord injuries, parents, educators, and students. Bowe felt sure the ADA could have profound effects, helping to reduce the budget deficit, alleviate the labor shortage, and energize the disability community. However, there was serious opposition from the National Federation of Independent Businesses and from transportation or-

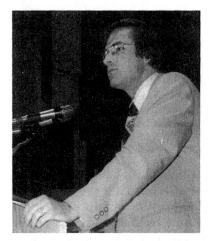

ganizations such as Greyhound. In an atmosphere of near- hysteria, fearing the costs of adhering to the new law, these well-funded special interests urged people to write to their elected officials and "stop the insanity." Fortunately, Frank Bowe and other advocates were ready, and could point with considerable authority to the experience of Sections 501, 503, and 504. Under these statutes, affected businesses prospered, and the costs of accommodations were demonstrated to be minimal.

Throughout the development of ADA, Frank Bowe's insistence on the inclusion of many important features resulted directly from his years of study, and experience in advocacy, international policy, and life as a person with a disability. First, Bowe maintained, it was critical that ADA *not* become an affirmative-action law. Groups protected by other civil rights laws (women, African-Americans, and other ethnic minorities) perceived goals and timetables as progress, but soon they regarded them as "quotas, which have the effect of reverse discrimination." Affirmative-action provisions were not consistent with the values Frank had developed while growing up in conservative central Pennsylvania. Worse yet, affirmative-action provisions were not politically viable, especially among conservatives in Congress and the White House. Frank Bowe felt certain that if they were included as a feature of the ADA, it simply would not fly legislatively. The ADA must emphasize non-discrimination and equal opportunity, but must not require preferential treatment.

To be successful, Bowe believed that the ADA must next have a balanced focus on cross-disability issues. By this time, Frank Bowe had become a bridge between the "deaf culture" movement and the independent living movement, two groups whose understanding and appreciation of each other had become strained. Frank Bowe was opposed to specialized services or protections for any single group. He believed that it was important for all disabled people to receive the same benefits and protections under the new law.

Frank Bowe's sense of humor and cross-disability bias were illustrated when he served as a panelist at a presentation sponsored by the American Federation of the Blind. At the scheduled lunch break, he offered his elbow to the federation's president to guide him to the men's room. On the way, Frank quipped, "This is a case of the deaf leading the blind." The story has been repeated many times in both communities.

Due in no small part to the involvement of Frank Bowe, the summer of 1989 was a "summer of compromise" among various advocacy groups, the

House, the Senate, and the White House. "By June of '89," said Bowe triumphantly, "I knew it was going to fly."

In July 1990, by overwhelming majorities, the House and Senate passed the ADA. With more than 3000 advocates, parents, and government officials in attendance, President Bush signed the ADA into law on July 26, 1990, on the south lawn of the White House. Frank Bowe was proud to attend. But mindful of his 504 experience, Bowe was just as eager to participate in the rigorous and thankless work of hammering out the regulations necessary to fully implement the law. Unlike 504, these were released in a timely fashion, one year after the signing ceremony.

Frank Bowe was concerned that the information age be as accessible as he hoped buildings would eventually become. From 1986 to 1988, Frank Bowe served as chair of the U.S. Congress Commission on Education of the Deaf. His 1988 report, *Toward Equality,* called for a federal law requiring the installation of a microchip in all new televisions to make them capable of generating captions. This way, deaf people, as well as foreign-born, young, or illiterate persons learning to read, could benefit. Frank Bowe went to the Far East to obtain support from the primary manufacturer of television sets. In cooperation with Senator Harkin, the final version of the ADA dropped the television captioning requirement. Harkin, whose brother was deaf, decided to pursue that issue separately, as PL101-431, the Television Decoder Circuitry Act of 1990. The law became effective in July 1993.

Issues of the day

There are other issues on Frank Bowe's plate these days. He believes the disability community needs to soon come to grips with a potentially frightening reality: America does not have the resources to continue the kinds of entitlement programs that many people with disabilities have come to depend upon, including Supplemental Security income (SSI) and Medicaid. In Frank Bowe's mind, these income redistribution programs, which, over the years, have guaranteed medical care and monthly checks, have been remarkably generous. During this same period, however, the nation has also invested billions of dollars to eliminate architectural, communication, and discrimination barriers, to give people with disabilities a better shot at the American dream. Says Frank Bowe, "Therein lies the conflict. On the one hand, society gives money to people who, Americans believe, cannot help themselves. On the other hand, society takes major steps to help these same people help themselves. At some point, voters are going to say, 'Enough! It's time for you to assume responsibility for your own lives.' "

Frank Bowe believes the time will come when entitlement spending will reach such a proportion of the overall federal budget that the American people will regard it as intolerable. Because he believes this point is inevitable, even imminent, Frank Bowe is alerting the recipients of these benefits, and the disability-rights community that this point will likely be reached soon. He is also working with the Social Security Administration and Congress to build more bridges to independence, such as vocational training and job placement programs, personal assistant services, and other transitional supports. Frank Bowe prefers this approach to the sudden and abrupt cut-off of current forms of support, which would inevitably result when the fund is bankrupt. Frank Bowe is trying to prevent a resurgence of homelessness, such as that which followed the deinstitutionalization of persons with mental illness in the 1970s and 1980s.

So, fifteen years after leaving Washington, D.C., Frank Bowe retains a "policy-wonk" mindset. He is among a handful of Washington advisers with a firsthand knowledge of national disability rights groups and thousands of individuals with disabilities. In meetings, conventions, and speeches he can listen and exchange ideas with stakeholders in these discussions. Their viewpoints are many and varied. What he sees and hears sometimes troubles him:

> I'm not sure how much the disability rights movement understands today's Washington climate. The independent living center directors, self-help group leaders, and others active in disability rights continue to see the federal government as a benevolent uncle, and they want more benefits, more services, more rights. But within Washington I see a very different picture. Most Congressional staff members with whom I work were not even there in 1990, much less in the 1970s when special education and rehabilitation laws were enacted. Members of today's Congress, mostly Republican, tend to view government as more of an enemy than an ally. It's going to be harder and harder to get good results out of Washington as the years go by. (Personal communication, 1997).

Frank Bowe believes that today the real promise for people with disabilities resides in the private sector. More disability-related services, communications products, assistive devices, and technological enhancements are emanating from there; most new job openings are to be found there; more of what matters on a day-to-day basis to people with disabilities can be found there. Frank Bowe remains optimistic:

> All of this means that policies on Main Street — company hiring policies, store accessibility policies, World Wide Web design policies — shape our lives in the 1990s as much as, and sometimes more than, policies on Pennsylvania Avenue in Washington. This, for many disability-rights advocates, is a strange turn indeed. Many still have the mindset that "business is bad" and "big business is even badder." These disability rights leaders are going to need to think all this

> through. If we want to make further progress in employment and in access to all that life has to offer, we may very well have to look to companies like Bell Atlantic, Citicorp, IBM, Microsoft, and many others as partners. In fact, if we do this right, these companies might carry over their pro-disability employment and product-design thinking to other countries, advancing the cause of people with disabilities worldwide. (Personal communication, 1997).

Practicing what he preaches, Frank Bowe has worked closely with a number of Fortune 500 firms, including NYNEX, Bell Atlantic, IBM, UNISYS, Xerox, and others. This consulting work, which began after he left Washington in 1981, has focused on human resources, public affairs, and public relations. He has also helped these companies develop accessible products using what is now known as "universal design" strategies. For example, he assisted NYNEX (a regional Bell operating company) in field-testing the VoiceDialing service, which was introduced in 1995. He helped them to be certain that this service, which lets people dial phone numbers simply by saying someone's name, is useable by individuals with unusual sounding voices, such as someone with cerebral palsy or Parkinson's disease.

A professional home

In the fall of 1988, Frank Bowe began to attend more to Dean Beilin's overtures to him to join the faculty at Hofstra University. The discussion with his family had been ongoing for nearly eighteen months, and Phyllis had been very encouraging, realizing that academia had always been a lifelong career goal for Frank. Located at Hempstead, Long Island, Hofstra is one of the nation's premier universities for accessibility. Hundreds of students with disabilities, ranging from cerebral palsy to muscular dystrophy, from deaf-blindness to specific learning disabilities, attend classes in full equality with 11,000 non-disabled students. The university's commitment to accessibility and to leadership in disability attracted Frank Bowe. In fact, as early as 1964, Hofstra's board of trustees had made a commitment to full-campus accessibility. Harold Yuker was the provost, an internationally known scholar in the measurement of attitudes toward persons with disability. Hofstra University was an institution that personified what Frank Bowe's professional life had been all about. In addition, several colleagues, including former NYU classmate Dr. Liora Pedhazur Schmelkin, now a professor at Hofstra, told him it was an excellent environment for teaching and scholarly work. He could not refuse this opportunity.

He joined the faculty at Hofstra University as a full professor in the department of counseling, research, special education, and rehabilitation. This new department was the result of a merger of several academic areas, all of which were familiar to Professor Bowe. Negotiating a full professorship at a prestigious university is no small accomplishment for an applicant without a previous academic appointment. However, Professor Bowe's experience, excellent publication record, and appeal to multiple disciplines within the department earned him precisely such a position. Tenure followed three years later.

As a professor, Dr. Bowe is known as an early riser who can always be heard pecking away at his computer. Students find him readily available and approachable for academic advisement or counsel. He teaches a full load of graduate courses, which he so enjoys that he has elected to teach year-round, including a special session that runs through the holiday season. This is unusual for full professors, many of whom are "burned out" on teaching and prefer to commit their time to more scholarly activity. Bowe is highly regarded by colleagues and students for his genuine commitment to people with disabilities, his depth of feeling, his commitment to family, and his exceptional teaching skills.

The reaction of students to Professor Bowe is described by colleagues as nothing short of fabulous. Noted for his high energy, he challenges his students, all of whom come to share his enthusiasm as the term progresses, mindful of his genuine concern for them. He is constantly updating and upgrading his materials, seeking feedback from students, regarding what they expect vs. what they receive. He relies upon his real-world experience and personal contacts to illustrate the legal and policy implications of every issue discussed. These contacts provide him with extraordinary credibility in the classroom, and represent a "value-added" dimension uncommon in most educational circles.

Taking nothing for granted, Frank Bowe continually strives to learn more about teaching, to improve his effectiveness, and to increase the accessibility of his instruction by soliciting accommodation requests from students whose impairments are unfamiliar to him. He believes that it is the *teacher*, not the student, who must initiate efforts to remove barriers to classroom communication. In spite of considerable recognition for excellence in teaching, Frank Bowe is never satisfied: "I'm still working at it." In recognition of the quality of his teaching and student advisement, Hofstra University in 1996 named Frank Bowe the University Distinguished Teacher of the Year.

Professor Bowe serves on many committees, and is rumored to give his interpreter an unsolicited break when the issues discussed are not compelling. In Frank Bowe's world, this is not daydreaming, but "selective listening." He is confident and politically savvy from his years on the Hill, yet outspoken at times. He is known for his clever, dry wit, practical jokes, and a periodic display of poignant cartoons. Professor Bowe does not shy away from administrative responsibilities. Indeed, although his academic roots are in the areas of rehabilitation and research, he coordinates the special education program for the department. In true interdisciplinary fashion, he successfully bridges the gap and rises above territorial interests to serve in the best interest of the university, his department, and the students. Special education is a large graduate program dedicated to preparing tomorrow's teachers of children and youth with disabilities.

Professor Bowe continues to produce as a scholar. He serves on the editorial boards of *Rehabilitation Education, Journal of Disability Policy Studies, Mental Retardation,* and other professional journals. He is the author of more than thirty-nine books — including two textbooks for graduate study — as well as scores of journal articles.

And one foot on the Hill

At Hofstra, Frank Bowe focuses on making the university as accessible electronically as it is architecturally. In his course on technology and disability, he explores issues of access to the computer and to communications in general. In 1996, he chaired a national conference at Hofstra on "Access to the Information Superhighway." As always, he recognized the potential national policy implications of the work he was doing. When Congress took up its long-delayed rewrite of the landmark Communications Act of 1934, Frank Bowe found himself at the center of negotiations once again. Shuttling between New York and Washington on an almost weekly basis, he worked with the House and Senate to ensure that the Telecommunications Act would do what the Americans with Disabilities Act had not done: make advanced communications technologies accessible to and useable by people with disabilities.

The Telecommunications Act, signed into law by President Clinton in February 1996, requires that virtually all new telecommunications products and services be accessible to customers who have disabilities. This includes cellular phones as well as the new digital phones that carry voice, data, and video signals. The Act also requires that most broadcast and cable television programming be captioned. The 1996 Telecommunications act requires that owners and distributors of television programming must caption their offerings, completing the loop begun by the television Decoder Circuitry Act of 1990, which mandated that most television sets must have the ability to display captions.

In 1997, Frank Bowe devoted his energy to the rewriting of federal laws which are critical to disability rights. These include the Individuals with Disabilities Education Act, the Rehabilitation Act, and the Education of the Deaf Act (which provides legislative authority and funding for Gallaudet College and the National Technical Institute for the Deaf in Rochester, New York).

Congressional staff members describe Frank Bowe as one of the key players in advocating for and enhancing the rights of people with disabilities. He gathers the facts, comes prepared, and fights hard for positive change. Yet he is both an advocate and a pragmatist, and therein lies his effectiveness. He is sophisticated in his understanding of the political realities involved in realizing a particular legislative objective. He appreciates the need to modify an approach, massage language, and compromise on portions of a bill, in the interest of moving it forward. Frank Bowe understands that it is this sense of reality that ultimately distinguishes a bill that makes an important statement from a statement that is heard as the bill becomes law. Along the way, his exceptional interpersonal abilities have functioned as a lubricant which keeps the entire advocacy machine in motion.

A day in the life

At his home on Long Island's south shore, and in his office at Hofstra, Frank Bowe's routine is dictated by the university schedule and the congressional calendar. He usually rises at 5:30 A.M., seven days a week. He finds the peace and quiet of the early morning hours to be conducive to his prolific writing. He reads and responds to dozens of e-mail and faxed messages each morning, then resumes his writing projects — books, articles, and the like. By mid-morning, it is off to the university where he handles administrative tasks, fields phone calls, advises graduate students, and performs committee work. Monday and Tuesday evenings are special — these are his teaching nights, and they are protected. Wednesdays or Thursdays, he can be found in Washington if Congress is in session; otherwise, these days are devoted to public speaking or advisory board meetings in the community. By Friday, Frank Bowe is back at Hofstra, doing library research or completing university administrative tasks. By late evening, he is at home with Phyllis.

Phyllis Barbara Schwartz grew up in Queens, the younger daughter of a middle-class family. Her mother, an employee of Air Canada, took her on frequent trips to Europe. Her father was a laborer, whose natural ability to design and build was overshadowed by his lack of opportunity for higher education. Her high school's valedictorian, Phyllis had a full and enjoyable upbringing, a sharp contrast to the isolation experienced by Frank.

> Phyllis has to put up with a lot. As a couple, we get invited to things like a jazz festival or a Broadway musical. Phyllis loves these, but because I am deaf she usually has to turn them down. When we go to movies at local theaters, she needs to sign to me so that I can follow along. When we go out to dinner with other couples, she has to interpret then, too. She has been amazingly patient about all these burdens, far more than I would have been had our situations been reversed. (Personal communication, 1997).

Phyllis Bowe is beautiful, graceful, intelligent, patient, and is everything Frank Bowe ever dreamed of in a partner. She shares with Frank a sardonic sense of humor. She is a movie fanatic whose ability to incisively dissect characters and their motivations adds to the enjoyment of movie-watching for Frank, who is making up for more than thirty years of life without cinema. The couple also plays tennis and reads — fiction for Phyllis and nonfiction for Frank. Phyllis is an interpreter and teacher at a local early-intervention and preschool special education program. As a front-line professional, she often learns about rare physical, mental, or emotional disorders, such as "-18Q Syndrome." Together, the two log onto the Internet and search for information. Thanks to Phyllis, Frank Bowe's own professional development has been even further enhanced.

Both Phyllis and Frank continue to be active parents to their daughters, Doran and Whitney, who are in college. Doran, who aspires to be an attorney, is completing her studies at the University of Pennsylvania, where she majors in creative writing and psychology. Whitney, a pre-med student at Yale, is a high achiever in science and mathematics. Frank looks forward to their visits home: "The girls are the lights of my life!"

The isolation and sense of "differentness" in Frank Bowe's childhood left him with some interesting personality features as an adult. For instance, there was considerable anxiety during his youth about whether or not "people like him" would ever be capable of earning a living wage. As a husband and father, he has no qualms about providing the best for the family in terms of "big ticket" items, although he is known for being careful with money. When shopping for groceries, Frank carries a shopping list that specifies exactly what brands to buy — otherwise he would bring home generic versions of everything. Frank will never use two paper towels when one will do the job. Ever the psychologist, Frank Bowe rationalizes that these idiosyncrasies are the logical extensions of his developmental fears. To Phyllis and the girls, he is just plain cheap.

In his "spare time," Frank Bowe serves on advisory boards for projects on universal design at the Trace Research and Development Center, University of Wisconsin, Madison, and at the Center for Universal Design, North Carolina State University. These projects focus on the design of telecommunications services, buildings, and home-use products. He continues to work on demographics with the U.S. Bureau of the Census, and with the Louis Harris and Associates polling firm. Previously, he was senior editor for TJ Publishers, a Maryland-based company that specializes in books on sign language and deafness. He served as chair of the advisory board for the Northeast Disability and Business Technical Assistance Center, a critical resource in the implementation of the Americans with Disabilities Act. He has also consulted for the World Rehabilitation Fund.

Frank Bowe has been selected for numerous honors and awards. He is named in *Who's Who in America; Who's Who in American Education; Who's Who in Public Relations; Who's Who in Computing;* and many other directories. He has received the Trustees' Achievement Award from Western Maryland College, the Career Achievement Award from the State University of New York at Albany, and the Distinguished Alumni Achievement Award from New York University. In 1991, the U.S. House of Representatives' Task Force on the Rights and Empowerment of Americans with Disabilities presented him with the Americans with Disabilities Act Award. In 1994, he was inducted into the National Hall of Fame for People with Disabilities.

In 1992, Frank Bowe received the Distinguished Service Award of the President of the United States, signed by President George Bush. In presenting this award, Justin Dart said:

> Frank Bowe has made independence fashionable. As the world's leading author on disability issues, he is the father of modern, independence-oriented disability policy. *Rehabilitating America* and *Handicapping America* have been the bibles of our movement.

Postscript

Reflecting on his first fifty years, Frank G. Bowe, Ph.D., professor at Hofstra University, waxes philosophical. Asked to name his greatest achievement, there is no hesitation, "Twenty-four years ago, I married the woman of my dreams. Phyllis has made me the man I am today." Pressed for his second greatest achievement, he promptly replies, "Raising two wonderful daughters, Doran and Whitney, and seeing them make so much of their lives."

Only then does he turn to the cornerstone of his own enormous reputation — federal legislation — from Section 504 of the 1973 Rehabilitation Act and the 1975 Individuals with Disabilities Education Act, through the 1990 Americans with Disabilities Act and the 1996 Telecommunications Act.

> You know, twenty-five years ago I set out to become a university professor. I finally made it nine years ago, and I am glad that I did. But the things I worked on in the interim, with so many others, have turned my professor life into an experience very different from what I expected a quarter-century ago. I never thought I would be living the life that I am now. I was 25 years old before I made my first telephone call; today, I make and receive dozens of calls every day. I always knew I could do good work, but I doubted whether anyone would give me a chance. In fact, the first time I asked for a job I was told, point-blank, 'We don't hire people like you.' Today, that would be illegal. To use the title of a book of mine, the rules have changed. (Personal communication, 1997).

Asked to describe his greatest frustration, he hesitates for the first time:

> This may be arcane for some people, but let me try. In 1972, before I got involved in Washington, Congress created an entitlement program assuring people like me a monthly check, virtually for life. It made some sense at the time. Certainly I was not the only one who

could not get a job offer in those days. Since 1972, however, we have made the country vastly more accessible. We have opened up educational opportunities I never dreamed of as a child, and we have made employment a realistic option for almost everyone who has a disability. We have changed the rules to give these opportunities to every American.

Yet millions of Americans with disabilities dismiss all the work we have done and opt to take those guaranteed checks every month. Some people with disabilities do need government entitlements. The vast majority, however, could do so much more, and live lives that are so much more meaningful and rewarding by grasping the opportunities we worked so hard to make available. (Personal communication, 1997).

Key publications by Frank Bowe

Bowe, F. (1995). *Birth to five: Early childhood special education.* Albany, NY: International Thomson Publishing Company, Delmar Publishers Division. A 600-page college and graduate school textbook.

Bowe, F. (1984). Access to the information age. *Policy Studies Journal*, 21(4), 765-774. A first-hand account of the intricacies of advocacy in the private sector involving disability rights groups and large corporations.

Bowe, F. (Ed.) (1991). *Approaching equality: Education of the deaf.* Silver Spring, MD: T.J. Publishers. This book, based upon a government report prepared by the Commission on Education of the Deaf (Chaired by Frank Bowe), led to major changes in education for deaf children, youth, and adults.

Bowe, F. (1986). *Changing the rules.* Silver Spring, MD: T.J. Publishers. Frank Bowe's account of his parents, growing up deaf, and his personal and professional development from the 1950s through the 1970s.

Bowe, F. (1981). *Comeback: Six remarkable people who triumphed over disability.* New York: Harper & Row.

Bowe, F. (1978). *Handicapping America: Barriers to disabled people.* New York: Harper & Row. One of the first books to lay out a social policy that encourages American society to take responsibility for the existence and removal of barriers to inclusion for people with disabilities.

chapter six

Tony Coelho

Robert T. Fraser

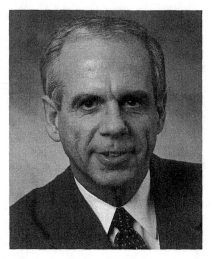

Former Congressman Tony Coelho: "Epilepsy shaped my destiny"

A middle-aged man with the easy bearing of an athlete twenty years younger moves across Philadelphia's 30th Street Station lobby toward the winged statue, which was our pre-arranged meeting place. Tony Coelho, the former Democratic powerbroker and Wall Street financier, was on his way to a management meeting at one of his New Jersey racetracks. Before the business trip, he was stopping to help me complete the story of his life. Tony is a man who these days is always looking for new challenges, as they can be "worked in." This is a man who wears an identifying epilepsy pendant on his muscular neck and who may be fingering his favorite rosary beads in his front pocket as he moves through the crowded station. His disability-related concerns, his commitment, and his spirituality, however, are never to be read as "soft" signs — these are core components of the man and have given him an unusual edge in every arena he has chosen to enter. Tony Coelho is undeniably a complex man, but the life impact of his Catholicism and his epilepsy are very clear. Although now primarily an east coast "mover and shaker," his developmental years and early epilepsy experiences began in the quieter milieu of California's San Joaquin Valley.

1-57444-083-7/00/$0.00+$.50

The early years

It's 3:00 A.M., and as young Coelho's alarm goes off, his work/school day begins. At a time when other twelve year olds are deep in slumber, Tony begins a "more-than-man-sized" day as he heads off to milk his family's cows and perform other farm chores before leaving for school.

Tony was born on June 15, 1946 in the farming town of Dos Palos in California's San Joaquin Valley. His family owned a dairy farm in a Portuguese farming community and Tony is a second-generation Portuguese. His mother's family had been dairy farmers, while his father's family had been fishermen. Tony learned about hard work and discipline at a very early age, working on the farm from the sixth grade until he left for college. The family's 300 cows required Tony to be involved in a very labor-intensive and rigorous milking schedule. He and his brothers and sisters worked from the time they got home from school at 2:30 until 7:30 every night. After that, he ate, studied, went to bed, and again was awakened at 3:00 A.M., in time to begin the cycle all over again. This schedule laid much of the foundation for Tony's disciplined approach to life.

The product of a strong Catholic family with a "killer" work ethic, Tony describes his mother as the "whip" in the family. As a young boy, he adapted to a blistering regimen of work. Unfortunately, much of the family's hard work turned out to be unnecessary, since his parents eventually went bankrupt after their sons went away to college or moved off the farm. They simply could not maintain the farm without help from their children.

There was, however, some limited time for fun. Tony remembers taking Sundays off and enjoying boating, attending the town's Santa Spiritu festivals, and going to evening dances whenever he could. In addition to the strong work ethic instilled by his family, he singles out his sixth-grade teacher, Dorothy Gould, as making him want to succeed and excel in life. She broached the idea of Tony pursuing a college education, and helped him develop his inner strength and a sense of purpose in targeting further educational goals. She was the first in a series of mentors who have guided Tony throughout his life. He seems to have a knack for both attracting mentors and then assuming that role for others.

Despite the various constraints on his high school time, Tony got involved in school activities and was elected student body president. He found a second mentor in the high school superintendent, Donald Bourne, who became a lifelong advisor. Bourne was always willing to listen and would meet with him almost daily to encourage him to set goals and to move out of the community to attend a good college. Bourne's mentoring during high school provided the spark Tony needed. He absorbed the concept that "failing is okay, but that it is important to believe in yourself and take a chance." Throughout his later years, he would drop by Bourne's home to discuss career moves and other issues. Bourne was always a part of Tony's "roots," as well as a "big-picture," future-oriented guide for him.

Tony's life took a dramatic turn at age fifteen, when a pickup truck in which he was riding flipped and he experienced a head injury that caused significant recurring headaches. His seizures started about a year later. These seizures tended to occur late in the day, about 5:00 or 6:00 P.M. He remembers them as being generalized tonic-clonic or "grand mal" seizures, as they were known in the old terminology. A neurological evaluation would later suggest that they were localized partial-complex seizures which, when not appropriately treated, generalized into the grand mal type of seizure. Partial-complex seizures by themselves generally involve a brief loss of consciousness and disorientation and often some automatic motor movements, such as clutching at clothing or brief wandering behavior. Although disconcerting, they can usually be controlled and are not as neurologically or physically impairing as a grand mal seizure, which involves several minutes of lost consciousness and full-body convulsions. His parents tried various medical clinics, herbal teas, and actual "witchcraft." To his Portuguese family, having epilepsy (from the Greek word for seizure) meant "possession by the devil." It was rumored within the Portuguese community that the ancestors of an individual with epilepsy had committed unnatural acts with animals. Punishment, therefore, was "divinely" forthcoming. The range of potential antidotes offered to Tony included pouring hot oil over his head, herbal treatments, and burning candles over him, each geared to driving out "evil spirits." One witch doctor complained that since Tony didn't believe in these treatments, he simply couldn't be helped. Consequently, while in high school, "treatment" for his condition ended with the witchcraft.

He states that at the time, "ignorance perhaps saved me," and "I decided it [epilepsy] really wasn't going to bother me and firmly compartmentalized it." Although his parents had been provided with a medical diagnosis of epilepsy, they simply would not accept it nor would they let Tony know specifically what he had. With this unclear medical issue in his life, and still being prone to an occasional seizure, young Coelho decided to leave town to attend Loyola University, a Jesuit university with a strong academic standing near the coast in west Los Angeles.

Despite their financial situation, Tony's parents managed to pay for college and he became very active in student government and politics. He was a member of Phi Sigma Kappa, a social fraternity. He thrived on working with diverse groups of people and liked being involved in a number of causes and issues. As a sophomore, Tony was the first non-local student to become class president. He became social chairman of his junior class, and as a senior was elected student body president. His political fund-raising skills were first honed at Loyola University. He made money for the student association through concerts by the Kingston Trio, the Beach Boys, and other groups. His goal was law school, until John F. Kennedy was assassinated. That terrible event had a profound impact on his life.

Tony describes himself as going into a "funk" for four days. He reassessed his priorities and felt that the loss of Kennedy positively influenced

him into "giving his life to others." Becoming a lawyer was now less important, and Tony's ultimate goal in public service switched from being a lawyer
to becoming a Catholic priest. Specifically, he wanted to be a Jesuit, the order
that had educated him in college and which had a reputation for theological
and philosophical leadership within the Catholic church. His girlfriend of
five years was shocked and upset, but his fraternity brothers understood his
commitment. As a graduate of Loyola University, and having been voted
"outstanding senior" and student body president, Tony could not imagine
a reason for not being accepted into the Jesuits. Life, however, was to present
a different turn of events.

Epilepsy makes a dramatic impact

A medical evaluation was a standard requirement as part of Tony's entrance
procedure into the Jesuits. On June 15, 1964, a local neurologist, Dr. John
Doyle, Sr., explained to Tony that he had epilepsy, a recurrent seizure disorder. He stated that, "The good news is that you don't have to serve in
Vietnam, but the bad news is that you won't be able to become a Catholic
priest — more specifically, a Jesuit." A section of the Roman Catholic
Church's 1917 Code of Canon Law stated that those with epilepsy, or "possessed by the devil," could not be considered for ordination. (Years later,
Tony led a delegation to the Vatican with an agenda to personally address
this issue with the pope, only to learn that it had been rescinded in the early
1980s.)

Dr. Doyle was very clear in his explanation of the disability. Tony felt
some immediate relief, as Dr. Doyle explained his disability using the anal-
ogy that "a tightly wound alarm clock" occasionally needs release. For Tony,
this "release" was a sporadic seizure incident. Following an emotional flood
of relief, the fallout began; it was clear to Tony that he was being rejected
by the Jesuits due to his disability. He then lost his driver's license and
insurance as a result of his medical diagnosis. But the most painful result of
Tony's diagnosis was rejection by his parents. While the diagnosis of epilepsy
was something they had known about for years, they had simply denied it.
In a phone conversation with Tony, the elder Coelho firmly stated, "No son
of mine has epilepsy!" Years later, Tony was able to reason that because
epilepsy was linked to "possession by the devil," and by superstition to other
negative family behaviors, accepting their son's disability would have
required acceptance of the belief by his parents that some family members
had committed grave sins.

Tony's life took a real slide. He had lost not only his desire for law, but
also his basic drive and motivation. He turned away from formal religion
because of its lack of acceptance. He felt that he had lost everything and
assumed that his friends had abandoned him. It was June in Los Angeles,
and he began hanging out in Griffith Park during the day, sitting on a hill
drinking wine. Suicidal thoughts entered his head and he contemplated
killing himself in an auto crash. He drove without a license, which he had

lost due to his epilepsy. Tony credits Hilda Crawford, a German immigrant and the mother of his best friend's girlfriend, with providing tremendous support by assuring him that "things would get better." Still, it seemed they couldn't be any worse. He felt that his God had rejected him, and spent days crying, truly feeling lost.

Through this period, his friend Jack Kane, with whom he had an intense love/hate relationship, also assisted Tony in several ways. He gave Tony a small pocket rosary, which he still carries in his front pocket. Jack, a former seminarian, also tossed him a novel entitled *Mr. Blue*, by Myles Connolly. The book made a very strong case about trying to understand yourself through the trials and tribulations of Mr. Blue, the story's protagonist. The book made a number of strong points that Tony has kept with him — the need to appreciate the little things in life, the fact that a friend can never take away from you what he or she has at one point given, the importance of not disempowering people by making life too easy for them (a mistake made when Mr. Blue comes into wealth), and a number of other axioms and messages that Tony utilizes in guiding his life to this day.

This was Tony's first real setback in life — he had overcome everything else with motivation and the investment of time. Finally, as Tony was sulking in Griffith Park one sunny day, the voices of children, laughing and shouting as they played on the merry-go-round, filtered through his glumness, touching something in him that he thought he had lost. He realized it was time for him, "just like these little kids," to believe, to trust, and to start over again. His Jesuit friends on campus had been supportive of him, but it was time for him to move on and embrace a new life direction instead of hiding and marginally subsisting in the old frat house.

Tony began to take the prescribed daily dosage of phenobarbital, which was the appropriate medication for epilepsy at that time (today he takes Tegretol). He felt the medicine helped, although he would occasionally be sleepy by mid-day. Tony realized that he may have lost supportive contact with his parents, but that the Jesuits were still there to assist him. Although their dogma had rejected him, they had not. He was determined not to allow himself to be dejected. It was time for him to find an area of service to others in which he could really contribute.

Bob Hope helps with a career and life transition

Through Father Ed Markey, Tony was recommended for work as a household aide to the actor and comedian Bob Hope. Although not Catholic himself, Hope's wife, Dolores, was Catholic and was very supportive of both the church and Loyola University. In addition, she had been voted Catholic Mother of the Year in the Los Angeles area. This was an exciting time for Tony, and it was also a time to think. He traveled with the Hopes and attended filming of the *Bob Hope Chrysler Comedy Hour*. Hope spent considerable time with Tony — occasionally driving the freeways with him simply to help him review potential service ministries in which Tony might get involved. Finally, Hope talked Tony into "the ministry of politics." Hope convinced Tony of the value of a public service ministry, and sent a letter to Bernie Sisk, a congressman from the San Joaquin Valley. At the time, Sisk needed an aide, and Hope's endorsement certainly helped. When Hope learned that Sisk had offered Tony the position of aide, he encouraged Tony to secure a loan from the Bank of America in North Hollywood for "start-up" funds for relocation to Washington, D.C. Through a bank administrator, Hope had already provided a "carte blanche" credit line for Tony. To Hope's surprise, Tony felt that all he needed was $1000 to establish himself in Washington. Although marginal, this amount allowed Tony to manage his basic needs, and on April 1, 1965, he moved first into a Washington, D.C. hotel and then into an apartment. He eventually became a key congressional aide to Congressman Sisk, whom he always referred to as "the boss." Since Sisk did not really understand agricultural needs, Tony gave him the agricultural acumen and edge that he needed to take on his "blue-blood" opponents who couldn't relate to the farmers' needs. He became a real asset to Bernie Sisk, and eventually he and Tony developed a father-son relationship. Tony had found another significant mentor, and became lifelong friends with Sisk and his wife.

Tony met his wife-to-be, Phyllis, in 1965 during Labor Day weekend. Phyllis was an aide to Representative Jacobs, a Democrat from Indiana. Although she did not have the college education he had always thought was important for his spouse, Phyllis was from the Midwest. Because of the strong midwestern values and clear thinking he had witnessed in a college classmate's mother years before, Tony felt that a Midwest birthplace was a positive attribute and was one of his criteria for marriage. With Phyllis meeting this key criterion, their relationship developed into a mutual bond of love and respect.

Concerns about his epilepsy arose for Tony when he decided to ask Phyllis to marry him. He felt obligated to tell her about his disability, an action which was very intimidating for him. He "didn't want to let anybody in on his secret," because he feared being emotionally rejected and hurt again, as he had been by his parents and the Jesuits. At a surprise party she gave for him, Tony ended up drinking too much and revealed his epilepsy secret to her, fully expecting rejection. To his surprise, Phyllis was more concerned about his getting drunk and had no problem accepting his disability. They were married in 1967, and Tony emphasizes today that she is not only his wife, but his "best friend." She has never had any difficulty accepting Tony's epilepsy, and has always provided the "rock-solid" base he felt he needed to pursue his goals in life. Phyllis was so unconcerned about his epilepsy that she never learned any first-aid* procedures. When she finally saw him have a seizure outside a restaurant, she protected his

---

* Basic epilepsy first aid would involve turning an individual on one side, clearing the area of debris to avoid injury, and timing the seizure — calling 911 or emergency assistance when a seizure exceeds five minutes in duration. The idea is not to call unnecessarily for a costly ambulance, but to seek help when seizures are not remitting within a reasonable period.

head, and actually put her finger in his mouth. This had no practical first-aid value, and was overtly dangerous — in this case, resulting in one painfully chewed finger. Although she now knows basic epilepsy first aid, she has seldom witnessed Tony's seizures — he has had less than ten in thirty-one years of marriage.

Phyllis has always admired Tony. She sees him as a very caring individual who is very sensitive to the needs of others. According to Phyllis, Tony can be confrontational and "tough on his friends, but only because he expects of them certain standards for themselves." Personally, states Phyllis, Tony is a very "humble man." Much of the time, Phyllis says, she has felt like a "minister's wife." "What a lot of people don't know," Phyllis says in an aside, "is that Tony can be a lot of fun" when he relaxes with friends, and that he really enjoys dancing. For a small-town midwesterner from Bedford, Indiana, life with Tony has been quite an experience.

Tony and Phyllis have two daughters. Nicole, an opera singer in Boston, also works for a law firm. Their younger daughter, Kirstin, graduated from the University of Richmond in Latin American studies and works in public relations for a bank.

Tony's success as an aide in Congress mounted steadily through the years from 1964 to 1977. He became Sisk's chief of staff, supervising twenty employees. He was the agricultural expert for Sisk's office and eventually assumed that role for the entire California delegation. He became a broker for agricultural legislation, establishing a niche for himself within Congress. He was also involved in a number of diverse subcommittees, including cotton, broadcasting, sports, and parking. Tony felt that Sisk considered him to be a partner on his team, and throughout Sisk's last five years in office, Tony believed he was being groomed to replace him. During those years, Tony's seizure "breakthroughs" were nearly nonexistent. In the early '80s, Tony tried to withdraw himself from medication, but after experiencing several seizures learned the hard way that this was not a good idea. He chalked this up to his ego and resumed compliance with his medication. Upon reflection, he was particularly chagrined by the fact that he could have been driving at the time of a seizure. For the most part, his epilepsy did not affect his day-to-day activities.

There was a day, however, when Tony, as member of a Washington, D.C. delegation that included Bernie Sisk, the mayor, and other city officials, flew to San Diego to attempt to purchase the San Diego Padres baseball team for the District of Columbia. On the plane, Tony had a partial complex seizure with secondary generalized convulsions. His associates loosened his tie, searched for his medication, and iced his forehead. Tony will never forget the group's respect and total lack of reaction or rejecting behavior. It confirmed his respect for his colleagues, and most importantly for his mentor, Bernie Sisk. In 1978, Sisk stepped down and gave Tony a chance to run for national office representing a district comprised of over fifty ethnic groups, which stretched within the San Joaquin Valley from Fresno to Modesto. The Sisks became lifelong friends of Tony and Phyllis, and Tony eventually performed the eulogies at their funerals. As a mentor, Sisk had prepared him well to run for Congress.

Tony's growth as a congressman and political "mover and shaker"

With Sisk's support, Tony ran for office in 1978, representing California's 15th district. He felt that he was progressing well in the race until his opponent raised the disability issue. His opponent questioned the impact that a "possible scenario" might have, in which Tony, while representing farming interests for the San Joaquin Valley, had a seizure in the middle of making a formal water-concerns presentation to the president. Tony's response to an inquisitive press seemed to win the day. Tony simply stated, "There are a number of people who present unique concerns and special needs to the president and leave the Oval Office having fits...at least I'd have an excuse!" This frank and humorous rejoinder was well received, and Tony won handily, garnering 62% of the district's vote. He had finally achieved membership on the floor of Congress.

Tony went on to serve five terms in Congress, and was elected to a sixth, from which he resigned in the summer of 1989. He and his staff built a highly organized and efficient political machine. Tony is generally perceived to be a firm taskmaster, yet he deferred to the expertise of his aides. He asked for frequent reports of his aides' activities and carefully critiqued their plans and accomplishments, often late into the night. He frequently turned over to an aide discussions between himself and a House colleague or business-person when he felt the aide was better versed on the topic. Tony considers his former staff to be family, and although he held them accountable for weekly progress memos and maintained an unyielding schedule, he was always available to help with their personal concerns and problems. He made sure each aide received feedback. He still holds annual get-togethers in the Washington area for several hundred former staffers, maintains a published directory of their whereabouts, and encourages their networking. He has former staffers in key positions within the House, the Senate, and the Clinton administration. Maintaining networks and promoting network development among friends is something at which Tony has always excelled. It is a natural outgrowth of his true commitment to people, his own experiences in being mentored, and his functional and expedient method of meeting personal goals, while promoting goal attainment for his colleagues. Tony's capacity to build and maintain networks of political colleagues, even across party lines, as well as former staffers, is still admired on the "Hill."

From 1981 to 1987, Tony functioned as chair of the Democratic Congressional Campaign Committee (DCCC). He was responsible for a ten-fold expansion of fundraising efforts and established the Harriman Communications Center, a multi-media communications and production center to nationally support Democratic campaign efforts. In the 1980 election cycle, the committee raised a paltry $1.2 million from a list of 13,000 donors. By the 1986 elections, under Coelho's leadership, the committee raised a record $15 million, and the donor base had increased to 300,000 names. He courted the business community — both through and outside of the Political Action Committee (PAC) structure, even crossing party lines on issues of importance, encouraging business people to donate to the Democratic party. Tony became a highly visible figure within the Democratic party. One of his close friends, Congressman Stenny Hoyer, reflected on Tony's years chairing the DCCC. Hoyer was running for a representative seat in Prince Georges County, Maryland. Tony was to school him in how to run a campaign and to provide funding support through the campaign committee. Stenny described an "initial clash of egos," but Tony's professionalism soon won his respect, and they became close friends. "The Republicans," stated Stenny, "had moved way ahead of us at that time." Tony's leadership and organizational moxie were greatly needed. Tony and Stenny Hoyer became friends for life. Tony's sensitivity and personal follow-up when Hoyer lost his wife will never be forgotten by the congressman. "Tony," says Hoyer, "has the capacity for extraordinary empathy."

Tony's organizational expertise and ability to focus on the party's needs brought the DCCC to state-of-the-art standards. Hoyer attributes Tony's success both to his attention to technical detail (e.g., mailing lists, media, working knowledge of diverse interest groups) and his ability to raise money or chair events that fill party coffers. Hoyer states that this whole effort was "truly superb" in its sense of vision and focus. It could only have been performed by someone like Tony, who is both "very bright," and yet "highly personable."

In 1986, Tony made appearances in more than sixty congressional districts in support of Democratic colleagues. Through his own PAC, the Valley Education Fund, Coelho had contributed more than $1.1 million to his fellow Democrats since 1985. This "leadership" PAC was one of the largest of its type in Congress. Tony was so successful with the DCCC that he was brought back by the White House as an advisor in 1994, during a period of party crisis. He again traveled throughout the country in support of his colleagues' and younger Democrats' campaign efforts.

From 1986 through 1989, he functioned as house majority whip, the third-ranking member of the House Democratic leadership. Tony took particular pride in having been popularly elected, and with his trademark attention to detail, personally verified and re-verified his votes among House Democrats, right up to the actual casting of the vote. His strategy was to get to everyone immediately and to contact them repeatedly. This included not only "those on the fence," but his own campaign manager, Representative Vic Fazio of California, and close friend Stenny Hoyer — with his attention to detail, no vote was assumed. He also quickly and tenaciously went after the voting supporters of other representatives as they "dropped out" of the race. After being elected house majority whip, Tony was very aggressive in the position. Within the House, he took on Speaker Tip O'Neill and the

Democratic house hierarchy whenever he felt that he and other younger Democrats needed more influence in the House.

While making dramatic political gains, Tony also devoted his energy to fund-raising for the needs of those with epilepsy. Tony had "come out" as an individual with a seizure disorder, and now as his political career took off, he made an increasing effort to financially support and push the initiatives of the Epilepsy Foundation of America (EFA). As a board member and Lifetime Director of EFA, he hosted a series of benefits and "roasts" for himself and benefits through which he raised millions of dollars for the foundation. At a roast in Washington, D.C., where more than $500,000 was raised for the Epilepsy Foundation's national employment programs at a $500-a-plate dinner, his sometime adversary, Tip O'Neill, called him "an unusually able, talented, and beautiful individual...I've never seen a man with the energy he has." Even Tony's Republican adversaries applauded his political tenacity and acumen. Jim Lake, press secretary for the Reagan-Bush campaign stated that "Tony is not going to let anything stand in his way...not his epilepsy, not his irreverent Republican friends. He's the toughest, sharpest adversary we have. I'm glad you're my friend...I just wish you were one of us."

Congressman Hoyer provides perspective on Tony's capacity to reach people. Hoyer states that Tony "competes hard," but truly makes "close friendships across party lines." Tony seems to be able to go toe-to-toe on issues without ever personalizing a battle. Hoyer states that he feels very personally connected to Tony, but that there are "at least fifty people who feel equally connected to Tony...so many people consider him a close friend."

The money continued to roll in to EFA's programs through Tony's efforts — not only for the development of employment programs at epilepsy affiliate organizations throughout the United States, but for public education and family support initiatives. In 1993, his "Kids on the Block" puppet show alone educated more than 70,000 people about epilepsy, most of them school children. The puppeteers were on the radio, and performances were scheduled on bicycle safety days, etc. More than fifty of EFA's affiliates have Kids on the Block puppets, thanks to funding from the foundation's Coelho Fund. The puppet program presents epilepsy information through carefully written dramatic skits, followed by question-and-answer interaction between the puppet characters that have epilepsy and the children. Children learn to demonstrate epilepsy first aid with the puppets after the performance. It is both a disability-sensitizing and educational experience for these grade schoolers.

The Americans with Disabilities Act (ADA): the acme of Tony's congressional career

Congressman Coelho had always been very open about his epilepsy disability. His increasing openness was further encouraged by EFA as he became more involved with the foundation. Through his involvement, he began to provide testimony to effect changes, specifically in relation to various archaic state laws, which negatively impacted individuals with epilepsy (e.g., the right to marry), and became nationally recognized as an advocate for individuals with his disability.

As a result of these public appearances, Tony was approached by Sandy Purino, a Reagan counsel on disabilities, and Roxanne Vierra, a member of the President's Committee on Employment of People With Disabilities. Roxanne's husband, Fred, was a principal officer of Telecommunications, Inc. (TCI), and they had a son with a disability. Although Tony didn't originally write the ADA bill, he was integrally involved in its refinement and assumed the responsibility for spearheading the bill through Congress. His good friend Congressman Hoyer helped him immensely on the House side. Tony was also helped when Senator Lowell Weicker submitted the bill on the Senate side. In order to make the strong bill more politically viable, its refinement initially required some negotiation with the community of people with disabilities and rehabilitation professionals. From 1987 until its passage, Tony labored to make this bill a major part of his legacy to the country and to those who must deal with disability on a daily basis.

From a strategic perspective, the bill was initiated in the Senate because there were seven subcommittees in the House that wanted to kill it. The bill was strongly embraced by Senator Orrin Hatch of Utah, a Republican who actually came to tears in its defense while trying to move it through the Senate. Senators Ted Kennedy, Tom Harkin, and Bob Dole were also instrumental in pushing the bill through. Overall, it moved through the Senate with relative ease.

Tony believed that, in addition to various subcommittees in the House of Representatives, the bill would face some opposition from the administration. John Sununu, President Bush's chief of staff, was opposed to the bill, as was Porter, his domestic policy adviser. Tony attempted an "end run" by making contact with President Bush directly, and he succeeded in establishing the president's commitment to the bill. President Bush had had a daughter with a disability who had died and Tony felt that his commitment was very sincere and relatively easily won. Within the House, there were a number of concerns. Tom Foley, the speaker, felt that the ADA as a law would come back to "haunt" Congress. Bud Schuster, the ranking representative in the Transportation committee, was very concerned. Schuster was well connected to Greyhound support and this bill was felt to have the potential for some very detrimental impact on the transportation industry. The strategy became to take it through some of the easier committees — first, education and labor — and then work through the more difficult committees: commerce, judiciary, public works, and transportation.

At this juncture, due to potential negative publicity and a possible investigation relating to a bond that Tony had purchased through Drexel Burnham Lambert, Tony decided to resign from the House of Representatives. President Bush, among others, called him on his birthday to congratulate him and to thank him for all his work through the years as a committed and astute public servant. Bush asked if there was anything he could "do for him" as he left office. Tony never hesitated. His response was, "I want to get ADA through." It was President Bush who ultimately turned the bill around twice, when blocked by administration officials Sununu and Porter, who didn't believe that the government should regulate work-related and other accessibility concerns for people with disabilities. As Tony states, "I needed to call in all my chits, not only from the president, but from other members of Congress in order to succeed in the Americans With Disabilities Act becoming a law." Tony truly is proud of the bill being passed, but is quick to emphasize that "the good news is the ADA has passed, but it's also the bad news." In sum, he continues to emphasize that we cannot sit on our laurels or relax — the implementation of ADA remains a continuing challenge within the workplace and our country at large. As other countries begin to embrace the spirit and legal thrust of this act, the challenge will become greater and truly international.

A career low point results in new opportunities

As previously mentioned, in 1989, Tony was accused of improper lending of funds used to purchase a $100,000 "junk bond" from Drexel Burnham Lambert. The allegation included possible use of monies from a campaign fund provided by Drexel for Tony's last election campaign. To purchase the bond, Tony had actually borrowed the money from a Democratic contributor who managed a savings and loan bank in Los Angeles, a loan that had nothing to do with campaign funds. Although he had repaid the loan in a timely manner, he (or his accountant) had neglected to disclose the loan, giving it the appearance of an impropriety — unfairly utilizing a political connection to make a profit. This was obviously fertile material for muckraking in the world of Washington politics. Tony had to quickly make a decision.

Rather than drag his family through a long, painful, and media-laden investigation, Tony decided to resign. This was not because he had done anything unethical. The loan for the bond purchase had actually been secured with part of his home equity. The bigger issue was that, understanding politics, he knew the tortuous procedures that would follow. He decided it was not in the best interests of the Democratic party, of the legislation that he was trying to shepherd into law, or in the best interests of his family to undergo the process. He would move on, clear his name through legal due process, and look for new challenges. His friend Congressman Hoyer urged him not to step down, as he was too much of an asset to his party. Family members, such as his daughter Nicole, were similarly distraught. Tony reasoned back that "everything I do could be second-guessed." It was time to go.

For most people, this would appear to be a very difficult step. Tony, however, with his typically clear thinking, simply saw the issue for what it was and never looked back. He describes a few poignant moments when one day in his garage, it occurred to him that he was walking away from several decades of committed political activities and a very prominent position within this country. The furor had subsided, and the reporters and colleagues were no longer around. Now the tears came and the pain swelled in his stomach — had he stepped aside too easily without a fight? The flood of emotions, however, subsided within twenty minutes. The anxiety left, the pain in his gut resolved, and he reassured himself that he had made the right decision. Several years later, Tony was exonerated of any unlawful or unethical activity. His legal defense, however, had generated almost $400,000 in expenses before the investigation was resolved. Tony felt that he never really experienced any emotional collapse. He still had his family, he believed that he had done nothing legally or spiritually wrong and had acted only in an honorable fashion, and within a matter of days, he had in excess of eighty private-sector job offers sitting on his desk. It simply appeared to be a time to look for new challenges. Phyllis looks back on those times with mixed feelings. It was an emotionally trying time, but she sees the period following this experience as the time when "we got our lives back." She couldn't remember Tony ever having a work-week evening dinner with the family while in Congress. The pain was replaced with an increased exuberance for life.

The leak of the information involving the loan could only have occurred through one of Tony's congressional friends, who denied responsibility. To this day, Tony does not understand his friend's motivation (e.g., jealousy, the opportunity for Tony's position, etc.). Although he never truly responded to Tony's confrontation regarding the leak, they remain good friends. His wife Phyllis attributes this to Tony's priestly orientation, bordering on the "saintly." Although Phyllis has a very strong set of personal values, even she can't get a full grasp on Tony's capacity for forgiveness. This is also part of his interpersonal philosophy, and harkens back to his reading of *Mr. Blue* during his formative post-college summer. Tony forgave his friend, in his heart, which has been his consistent orientation with others.

The former congressman tackles Wall Street

One of the offers made to Tony after his resignation from Congress was to become a partner or managing director at the New York-based international investment firm Wertheim, Schroder, and Company, Inc. When Tony came on board, the firm was struggling with a steady dwindling of its investment base. Steven Kotler, then forty, a former managing director, executive committee member, and head of investment banking for the company, was made president. His vision was to build a team that would restore the company to its former heights. Tony had been introduced to the company by James Lake, a former aide to Tony who actually had very strong Republican ties (e.g., former communications director at the 1988 Republican National Convention). Tony had initially met with Kotler while raising money for his epilepsy programs, and Kotler recalled him as a highly motivated and capable individual. He believed that the managerial skills that made Tony successful in Congress could be directly and successfully applied to the company. Within a few months of his hire, the former congressman was made chief operating officer of the firm's new investor-services subsidiary. Kotler, the company's president, challenged Tony to assist in turning things around. The investment base was $400 million and losing ground. Kotler also challenged Tony to acquire a real understanding of the business marketplace. He offered him a $100,000 annual bonus to read the *Wall Street Journal* from cover to cover every day, as part of a "crash course" in finance.

Tony was a quick study. His organizational acumen, superior interpersonal skills, and network of national contacts served him well. He deftly divided his time among asset management, the development of corporate accounts, and the firm's marketing and public relations efforts. In four and a half years, the company's asset base grew to $5 billion. Tony had brought into the Wertheim Schroder fold national players and unions such as the Communications Workers of America and the International Brotherhood of Electrical Workers. They "stayed," not simply due to a standing association with Coelho, but due to the firm's superior fund performance. Tony's attention to detail, his tirelessness, his goal-setting, and computer system upgrading were all making a difference. There was no looking back on his political career.

In January 1990, Tony was appointed president and CEO of the company. He began to serve on several corporate boards. In 1994, as the company moved toward a merger with Tony scheduled to direct a new investment-bank division, he paused for thought. The company had offered Tony $2 million a year for each of fourteen years, plus bonuses. He had enjoyed the Wall Street experience, he reveled in his establishment of a five-year plan and the setting of significant financial goals for the firm, but he was uncomfortable with being assigned a more structured role within the merger. Tony had achieved the financial security he needed for his family and his children's education. It was time to move on. Regretfully, he told Steve Kotler of his decision, and in October 1994, he launched his own business.

In a short amount of time, he was asked by Telecommunications Incorporated (TCI) to jump-start their new subsidiary, Educational Technology and Communications (ETC). Tony was up to the challenge. Over several years, he built the new company into a highly profitable operation which provided high-quality educational software, increasing the company's size from seven employees to over five-hundred. In the spring of 1997, ETC was sold. The sale of the company by the parent company, TCI, resulted in another substantial financial gain for Tony, but he was again left with the challenge of finding a new direction.

New challenges from the President's Committee

With the development of ETC in the Washington, D.C. area, Tony had found himself spending more time in the capital, and in March 1994, President

Clinton appointed him chair of the President's Committee on the Employment of People With Disabilities. John Lancaster, the current executive director of the committee, states that Tony, the "big-picture strategist," brought
about some "amazing changes." At that time, the agency was in considerable
disarray with forty-one initiatives under a "vague white paper" template.
Tony made new appointments to the board, resulting in an effective blend
of national employers, labor leaders, representatives from veterans' and
advocacy organizations for those with disabilities, media representatives,
and members from regional/federal government. The impact on his staff
was immediate — a number of staff changes occurred and Lancaster was
recruited for the executive director position after a new job was secured for
the incumbent director. The goals of the organization became organizational
clarity and discrete outcomes.

Today, the President's Committee has a streamlined look, with twelve
tightly managed projects having specific goals and measurable outcomes
within a targeted budget. Outreach to neglected disability groups (e.g., those
with psychiatric or learning disabilities) has been undertaken. The vagueness
in direction has disappeared, replaced with such specific projects as employment partnerships with the private sector, workday telecommuting for people with disabilities, strong support for the national Job Accommodation
Network at West Virginia University, and self-employment or small business
emphases for people with disabilities. The High School High Tech Program,
which links technology to student needs, is resulting in paid high-tech internships for students with disabilities. Presently, there are twenty of these sites,
with three to four being added annually.

Lancaster notes that all professional staff members are responsible for a
monthly report to Tony while he communicates in one phone session per
week with his executive director. "Some staff find his phone sessions rather
brusque," states Lancaster, "but I love them because Tony is a clear commu-
nicator and I get more done in minutes than in hour-long meetings." There
appears to be no question about Tony having provided a sense of purpose
and clear direction to an organization that had been having difficulty maintaining a substantive course of action. Tony has truly "brought home" to the
Clinton administration the employment concerns of people with disabilities.
Lancaster cites the development of the Presidential Task Force 2002, the
Employment of Adults with Disabilities, and Tony's vice chairmanship of
this task force as further examples of Tony's concerns about high unemployment for people with disabilities.

Where does Tony go from here? — An issue of balance

Today, there are a number of thoughts in Tony's mind relative to new roles.
It is obvious that no "moss" will grow beneath his feet. Tony has become a
majority owner, with partners, of two racetracks in New Jersey and a casino
in Las Vegas. He is actively involved in a number of corporate boards,
including Kistler Aerospace, TCI Service Corporation, Kaleidoscope Inter-

national, ICF Kaiser, and Cyberonics where he serves as chair or vice chair on several boards. He serves as board chair for the International Thoroughbred Breeders Association. Tony is particularly enthusiastic about his board activity with Cyberonics, makers of the vagal-nerve stimulator, a device having a significant impact on seizure reduction for many individuals with epilepsy. He has been recruited, "on the side," with several other northern Virginia businessmen, to attempt again to bring baseball back to the greater capital area. It would be difficult to find an individual with more diverse business interests.

The former congressman has also not entirely distanced himself from political or governmental assignments. He had been a Democratic appointee to the U.S. Census 2000 Monitoring Board. President Clinton also appointed him as Ambassador to Expo in Lisbon, Portugal. Tony felt that he could handle these "off-shore" responsibilities during one week per month. The question might be "involving how many hours in the week?"

Tony is a product of his Portuguese ethnic background, his "driven" family work ethic, his Catholic world view, and the sense of purpose provided by his epilepsy. All of these variables operate upon him in a manner that pushes him to new challenges in both the corporate "for-profit" and the "non-profit" arenas. Every ounce of his energy is put into life's fray on a daily basis — being productively busy is an elixir and there are no boundaries between work and leisure. His only known hobby is weightlifting: an activity consuming two-and-a-half early morning hours, five days per week. In his mid-fifties, he can easily bench press thirty pounds more than his 165-pound frame. His workouts are as "built-in" as his Catholic faith is. Today, Phyllis is thrilled with the time they have recouped and with the enjoyment of their homes in Old Alexandria, Virginia, and Bethany Beach, Delaware. Their time at the shore is particularly precious to both Phyllis and Tony.

The former congressman has taken on the challenge of the private sector and has succeeded in an impressive manner. In his embracing of the private-sector challenge, had he forgotten his mission to serve those with epilepsy and other people with disabilities? One supporter obviously thought so. Within the last year, he received a letter from a "fan" with epilepsy who had followed his career. The "fan" accused the former congressman of turning his back on the epilepsy community due to the enticements of the private sector. This was hard for Tony to swallow — didn't he still serve as a director of the National Organization on Disability, the National Rehabilitation Hospital and other meaningful non-profit organizations (e.g., National Foundation for Affordable Housing Solutions, and Very Special Arts)? Tony re-read the letter, again disputed it to himself, but left it on the side of his desk. After several weeks and additional "re-reads" of the letter, Tony contacted the Epilepsy Foundation to increase his involvement. He has now become further invested in both advisement and fund-raising. Maybe this supporter had something. He would put meaning into his appointment as a lifetime director for the Epilepsy Foundation. His constituency with epilepsy would never be forgotten.

Conclusion

As Tony left the presidency of ETC in 1997, he thought that this might be his time for reflection, to pick and choose his next course of action. He stated that he still wanted to be a "priest" if he could. Perhaps a satisfying pursuit might be a career as a chancellor in education, an ambassador down the line, or another direction in which he could truly contribute, on a national or international basis.

It now appears unlikely that Tony will have this "retreat" time to set his personal and individualized direction. The private and public service sectors keep knocking on his door with new opportunities and responsibilities. Other than his early morning workouts, leisure must be incorporated into the diversity of his business and public-advocacy activities. There is no question that epilepsy "acted upon" Tony Coelho. It has shaped him, strengthened him emotionally, and guided him, along with his Catholicism, toward public service for the good of his political district's residents, the Democratic party, and the public, both within and outside of the rehabilitation community. Tony says that "I will always be committed to making a difference...we have very little time on this earth." At this juncture, he maintains a balance in his time, invested between business and the rehabilitation community's needs and interests, a balance reinforced by the presence of the epilepsy medallion hanging from his neck and the feel of his favorite rosary beads in his front pocket.

Appendix A

A call to revolution

An agenda for Campaign 2000
Democracy goes on the offense
America for all: a revolution of empowerment

Americans, colleagues, you have created miracles of progress and promise for people with and without disabilities. Thanks to patriots past, thanks to you, America is the richest, the most democratic nation in history. The economy is at a record high. Crime is down. The federal deficit is gone. Starting with almost nothing, you of the disability community have established a great beginning foundation of basic rights to access virtually every aspect of society. We humans finally have the resources to eliminate discrimination and poverty, to remove the underlying causes of hate, crime and war.

But we seem unable to keep the promise to all. In the midst of record American prosperity, the poverty gap continues to grow. Millions of lower income workers struggle unsuccessfully to achieve the minimum standards of living with dignity in our society. There are millions with inadequate food, housing, health care. In other lands starvation, genocide and war abound. In spite of the historic victories of our movement, people with disabilities everywhere are still the oppressed of the oppressed.

Powerful political forces attack democracy. They pander to our addictions to the primitive values of our long predemocratic childhood under authoritarian paternalism. They prey on our fears of change, marketing massive escapism. They promote our prejudices, setting us off one against another. They attempt to destroy the democracy for all envisioned by Thomas Jefferson, Abraham Lincoln, FDR, Martin Luther King and Bill Clinton. They would lead us back to the days of power and privilege for the few.

They killed universal health care, the Patient's Bill of Rights and the Jeffords-Kennedy Bill. They attacked the ADA in 1990 and they attack it now. They attack the IDEA, Social Security, civil rights, affirmative action, clean environment, gun control and the freedom to make one's own choices about sex, religion and childbirth. They block MICASA and the expansion of community-based services. They attempt to cut taxes for the rich and reduce investments in the people. They attempted to impeach the President who has led America to its greatest days and who has empowered people with disabilities in his administration as never before. They plan to take the White House in 2000.

Congratulations to all who have defended democracy.   You have held the line for justice — ADA, IDEA, the FDR memorial, the '96 and '98 elections, Jeffords-Kennedy, the impeachment and much more. We have progressed in a few areas, but in most we are on the defense, in some we are in retreat. The time of miracle progress is over. Millions of people are still left out of the dream. Democracy is on the defense. Democracy is at risk.

A frustrated majority of Americans hunger for a practical vision of a society with responsibility for all. We have that vision.

> Now is the time for democracy to get off of the defense and onto the offense. We must convince others who love the human dream to join us in a revolution that empowers all to live their God-given potential.

- A revolution that replaces addictions to primitive symbols of power and exclusivity with that most profound power of love for the quality of each life and of all life.
- A revolution to create a new culture that focuses the full power of science and free-enterprise democracy on the systematic,, individualized empowerment of every person.
- A revolution that empowers all people to live their full potential to govern self and society, to produce the best possible quality of life for self and for all.
- A revolution that educates families, advocates, providers of services to create empowering environments for children and others who may not be able to make all of their own decisions for a period of time.

Only this profound revolution will carry us to our goal: a world of love, dignity, peace and the good life for all.

The word is all.   Until all people — people with and without disabilities, rich and poor, young and old, minorities and majorities are empowered to participate fully in the struggle for the good life, the promised land, the truly good life, will not exist. Only an aggressive politics of America for all will unmask the enemies of democracy by contrasting their elitism with the true goal: "All."

America for all. A draft platform for a revolution that empowers all.

Government by all: Government by you. Government by us. Government by every individual. You, we must take full responsibility to create and to be government that empowers all. We must provide the specific supports that will empower each person to govern self and society.

Responsibility for all: We must reconstruct tax codes so that all will pay their fair share. We must substantially revise the budgets of government at all levels, cutting the fat, the deficits, the bureaucracy, the special subsidies for the power elite and greatly expanding investment in empowerment services. We should consider requiring public service for youth and adults, with individuals making the final decisions about how they will serve.

Human rights for all: We as government at all levels must mandate and enforce the inalienable right of every person — with or without a disability — to live, to live free, to be protected from restraints and assaults on body and dignity. No assisted death.

Equal opportunity for all: We must mandate and enforce the inalienable right of all people to have full, equal and effective choices to participate in every aspect of culture. We must act affirmatively to protect, enforce, and strengthen the ADA and all civil rights laws. Gays, lesbians and others must receive full protection.

Health care for all: We must guarantee that all people receive comprehensive, quality, lifetime health care that empowers them to choose their doctors and treatments. All necessary health services must be covered, with no inflexible financial limits and with no forced treatment. The rationing of health care is not an option of civilized society. We must use intensive education and technology to empower all people to be the senior partners in their health care relationships — to provide simple services in the home. We must establish and enforce strong guarantees of patients' rights, including the right to take legal action when injustice occurs. For the short run, we must defend and strengthen Medicaid and Medicare and other empowering health care programs at the national, state and local levels.

Real choices for all: We must guarantee to each person lifetime free choice access to all the resources of the culture, including consumer-controlled services provided in the most integrated settings. We must empower all people to live and participate in their communities in ways that are voluntary and freely chosen. Let the values of independent living govern the culture. Let no American ever again suffer enforced isolation in an institution, a nursing home, a back room or any other place. Each person is entitled to, each person must be enabled to create and continually develop, a package of individualized public and private empowerment supports. This system must encourage and strengthen the dynamic diversity of our culture. We must transcend coerced conformity to stereotypical categories and provide real free choice for all. There will be no categories, no cracks to fall through. You qualify by being human.

Education for all: We must guarantee birth-to-death education, including higher education, which enables all individuals to choose from among the entire spectrum of public and private information resources. Universal, lifetime education is absolutely necessary in an age of exploding change and complexity. Parents, youth and adults must be empowered to construct individualized educational packages that include far more internships in the public and private sector. We must protect and strengthen the IDEA and other initiatives that guarantee first-class mainstream education to all.

Employment for all: We must guarantee lifetime services that empower all individuals to achieve their full potential for employment — decent jobs with decent pay, decent standards of living and decent opportunities for advancement. We must strengthen the Rehabilitation Act, creating a program that provides full choice, consumer-controlled services for all who need them.

Dignity for all: We must guarantee lives of dignity for all. We must reconstruct Social Security and other social-support programs to eliminate disincentives to work, to create programs that encourage all people to be productive and at the same time guarantee lives of quality for all who can't work or who are working but cannot earn a living wage. Cuts in SSI payments to children with disabilities must be restored.

Housing for all: We must work with the private sector to guarantee all individuals affordable, quality and accessible housing. All housing must be of universal design.

Life can be a Superbowl where everyone wins.

Communications and technology for all: We must guarantee all individuals practical, affordable access to all communication systems and other technology. We have the technology to turn every living room into a workplace, a university, a theater and a one-stop shopping center for public and private services.

Transportation for all: We must guarantee public and private transportation. that is affordable, accessible and available to all. There should be greatly increased investment in efficient, accessible public transportation, not only in large cities, but in suburban and rural areas. Owning and driving an automobile should not be required in order to participate in mainstream society.

Communities for all: We must join with the private sector to develop entirely new communities that are efficient and accessible as a whole — communities where all public places and services will be completely affordable, convenient and accessible to all people. Communities where you can get where you are going in a few minutes instead of a few hours. We built the shopping center. It's time to build the living center.

A world for all: We must empower the United Nations to enforce the letter and the spirit of their Standard Rules on disability and to become an aggressive force for the empowerment of all people. We must provide political, technical and economic support for the empowerment of people in every nation. Every representative of American government and business and every American tourist should be an ambassador of empowerment.

America for all! You have the power. Lead!

We can win, if you lead, if you can convince a few others to act. You have the power and the responsibility to lead the revolution that will save democracy and empower all people to live the human dream. You don't need any title or permission to act. Our message: *You can become a revolution of one — today* — in your own living room and community. Reach out to your family, your friends, your government and especially your colleague advocates. Your action will change society immediately because you are society.

> Let us unite to shout, "People of America, people of
> the world, you have power! Join us in the revolution
> to empower all."

Become a politician for empowerment.

- Pursue a politics of action. There is an action role for everyone, from civil disobedience to civil service, from recruiting your mayor to recruiting your mother. Power is never given. It is taken by people with the will to act.
- Pursue a politics of solidarity with all who love justice. Join, support, contribute to their organizations and their political campaigns. United we win. Divided we lose.

- Pursue a politics of simple truth. Leave deviousness to the demagogues. Truth is a magic sword for positive change.
- Pursue a politics of adamant persistence. History proves that you cannot beat people who simply refuse to lose. That is the real secret of winning: you never, never, never give up.
- Pursue a politics of love. Love is the ultimate power to reach hearts and minds, to change lives. All people are potential allies. Attack the bad idea; love the person.
- Pursue a politics of now. Every day is action day. Every day is election day. Those who wait for the official campaign and voting days severely limit their impact. The elections of 2000 are being decided now. Form an America for All group in your community today.

The world is watching our movement; the world is watching America. The world will follow what we do. Failure is unthinkable. Fight for empowerment as if your lives depended on it. They do, and the lives of all humans in the 21st century.

Let us embrace and lift each other. Let us reject hostility, self-indulgence and retreat. Let us go forward together in the great tradition of Jefferson, Lincoln, Gandhi, Martin Luther King, Nelson Mandela, Ed Roberts, Wade Blank and Elizabeth Boggs. Let us meet intimidation with courage, hate with love, demagoguery with simple truth. Let us overwhelm fear and fallacy with our positive vision. Let us unite to shout, "people of America, people of the world, you have power! Join us in the revolution to empower all."

America for all! You have the power. Act today!

1. *Form an America for All 2000 campaign today in your living room, in your community, in your state.* You don't need by-laws, titles or anyone's permission. If necessary, you can be a revolution of one.
2. *Volunteer regularly for good campaigns.* You can become an early leader in the campaigns of candidates and parties most likely to support the America for All agenda. Work in their offices. Attend their meetings with your America for All signs. Knock on doors. Pass out literature in malls. Contribute money — even a small contribution, will put you on a different list.
3. *Recruit family members, friends, business, church and advocacy colleagues to support the America for All campaign.* Don't be discouraged if there are only a few in the beginning. Those who attack democracy have made the politics of all seem unattainable. Remember, the Christian religion was started by 13 penniless people who didn't even have a room to meet in.
4. *Reach out to, join, support groups that may become strong allies for America for All.* Civil right groups, churches, advocacy groups, professional

groups, independent living centers, disability coalitions, ADAPT, DREDF, CCD, NCIL, TASH, ACB, NAD, Speaking for Ourselves, psychiatric survivors and many more. The will have their own specific agendas. But if you support them, they will support you. You will be able to convince some of their members to act as individuals in support of good political campaigns — at the very least by lending their private names.

"Colleagues, we love you!
Together we shall overcome!"

Justin and Yoshiko Dart

Appendix B

National Disability Policy: A Progress Report

Prepared for the National Council on Disability, Marca Bristo, Chairperson

Last Updated February 16, 1999

The views contained in this report do not necessarily represent those of the Administration, since this document was not subjected to the A-19 Executive Branch review process.

Preface

The National Council on Disability (NCD) is an independent federal agency charged with advising the President and Congress on public policy issues affecting people with disabilities. Consistent with this mission, NCD is required to report annually on the progress made in federal policy for people with disabilities and to make recommendations for how public policy might better meet the needs of the disability community. Given the diverse nature and large size of the disability community and the range of public policy issues affecting this community, NCD has tried to focus on issues that could affect large segments of the disability community in the United States.

As indicated on the title page, the following report covers the period from November 1, 1997, through October 31, 1998. NCD assesses developments in multiple areas of public policy against the yardstick of NCD's previous reports and recommendations. The principal report that forms the framework for NCD's policy analysis is its 1996 report, *Achieving Independence*, which captured the consensus recommendations of a diverse group of over 300 disability leaders from around the country who gathered in a summit in Dallas that year. To assist the reader, the following report below

1-57444-083-7/00/$0.00+$.50
© 2000 by CRC Press LLC

uses italics for text that includes NCD's recommendations for the President and/or the 106th Congress.

Introduction

On July 26, 1990, when he signed the Americans with Disabilities Act (ADA) into law, President George Bush said:

> ADA is powerful in its simplicity. It will ensure that people with disabilities are given the basic guarantees for which they have worked so long and so hard. Independence, freedom of choice, control of their lives, the opportunity to blend fully and equally into the right mosaic of the American mainstream.

President Bush later stated, "When you add together federal, state, local and private funds, it costs almost $200 billion annually to support Americans with disabilities, in effect, to keep them dependent." As President Bush recognized, the dependence-oriented model of our systems of public income supports and corresponding health care benefits is not consistent with ADA's vision of freedom of choice and equal employment opportunity. If you must lose your health care and personal assistance services when you take a job, is that equal employment opportunity?

In an effort to address in our public disability benefit programs the ongoing barriers to work, members of Congress engaged in a bipartisan, bicameral strategy this past year to allow people with disabilities to leave the disability benefit rolls and maintain their health coverage when they take a job. Another important component of the strategy would have expanded access to private vocational rehabilitation for people on the Social Security Disability Insurance (SSDI) and Supplemental Security Income (SSI) rolls. The return-to-work bills captured the attention of people with disabilities, their families, and advocates across the country as news of them arrived by e-mail, facsimile, telephone, and letter. Through the hard work of disability advocates and the bills' chief sponsors, the Ticket to Work and Economic Self Sufficiency Act in the House and the Work Incentives Improvements Act in the Senate gained the support of the Administration and almost became law. The progress made on this issue in the 105th Congress will form a solid foundation on which to build a successful bipartisan effort in the 106th Congress.

Independent of the return-to-work effort, reform of the Social Security and Medicare programs will be high on the list for both parties in the 106th Congress. As with other high policy priorities such as school modernization, managed care reform, physician-assisted suicide, or the implications of the human genome project, the manner in which Social Security solvency and the future of Medicare are resolved will have a great impact on people with disabilities. And yet, despite this, too few working-age people with disabilities and their advocates have participated in the ongoing discussions about how to protect the solvency of the Social Security Trust Fund or the future of the Medicare program. As more people with disabilities, their families and advocates speak out on Social Security and Medicare issues, the challenge they face will be defending the existence of basic federal income support programs and publicly funded health care coverage for those unable to work, while at the same time pushing for expanded access to affordable health and long-term services and supports for people with disabilities who seek employment. This challenge is present in many areas of public policy today. Should people with disabilities fight to protect important but poorly designed and poorly managed public programs as these programs come under heightened scrutiny, or should they proactively work to modernize public programs so that work and economic self-sufficiency will truly be promoted?

President Clinton recognized the need to modernize and coordinate federal policy to promote employment of people with disabilities on March 13, 1998, when he signed an executive order establishing a National Task Force on Employment of Adults with Disabilities. He named Labor Secretary Alexis Herman as chair and Tony Coelho of the President's Committee on Employment of People with Disabilities as vice chair. In the National Council on Disability's (NCD's) 1996 report *Achieving Independence*, which summarized the recommendations from a summit attended by a diverse group of over 300 disability community leaders from around the country, NCD recommended that the President sign an executive order directing the secretary of labor to promote the employment of people with disabilities by establishing national goals. This recommendation was expanded upon by political appointees with disabilities throughout the Administration and ultimately became the executive order signed by President Clinton in March 1998.

As stated in the executive order, the purpose of the task force "is to create a coordinated and aggressive national policy to bring adults with disabilities into gainful employment at a rate that is as close as possible to that of the general adult population." This high-level task force includes Herman, Coelho, the secretaries of education, health and human services, treasury, commerce, transportation and veterans affairs, as well as the commissioner of Social Security, director of the Office of Personnel Management, chair of the Equal Employment Opportunity Commission, administrator of the Small Business Administration, and the chairperson of the National Council on Disability. The task force has been working in subgroups in preparation for a November 1998 report to the President. After it issues the report, the task force will begin to solicit input from the disability leaders on preliminary recommendations and further directions for the task force. Like the President's Initiative on Race (PIR), the Task Force on Employment of Adults with

Disabilities provides an opportunity to educate all Americans about why people with disabilities have such low employment levels and what it will take to increase employment of this population. Equally important, the existence of the multi-agency task force signifies that the issue of employment of adults with disabilities is not simply a matter of vocational rehabilitation but instead requires a systematic revamping of the public and private systems that children and adults with disabilities must navigate successfully to get and keep a job.

One system that must be navigated successfully to get to work is the transportation system. The Department of Transportation (DOT), which has been an active participant in the work of the Presidential Task Force on Employment of Adults with Disabilities, took an important step this past year to making intercity travel more accessible and affordable for travelers with disabilities when it issued its final rule on over-the-road bus accessibility. This requires every new bus purchased by a major carrier after the rule's effective date to be fully accessible for travelers in wheelchairs. The rule also requires full fleet accessibility over time as old buses are replaced with new ones.

Like transportation, home- and community-based personal assistance services must be available and affordable for working-age people who need assistance with activities of daily living to find and keep employment. With a well-attended March 1998 hearing on the Medicaid Community Attendant Services Act (MiCASA) in the Health Subcommittee of the Commerce Committee, Congress this year received eloquent testimony on the need for legislation that would provide real choices in the community for children, adults, and seniors who need long-term services and supports. This legislative effort also was buttressed by a July 1998 letter from the Health Care Financing Administration (HCFA) to state Medicaid directors informing them of the ADA requirement that Medicaid-financed services, including long-term services, be provided in the "most integrated setting" appropriate. These two developments may be harbingers of broad-based efforts in the next Congress to eliminate the institutional bias in the current system and give people with disabilities and their families the ability to choose where to live and where to receive the long-term services and supports they need.

The return-to-work bills, President Clinton's Executive Order on Employment of Adults with Disabilities, the over-the-road bus regulations, the MiCASA hearing, and the HCFA letter all point toward progress in public policy; however, the last year also witnessed attempts to move the country backward by weakening civil rights protections for children with disabilities and their families under the Individuals with Disabilities Education Act (IDEA). Dissatisfied with the compromise on discipline that had produced sufficient votes to reauthorize IDEA in 1997, powerful members of Congress sought to amend the new law to make it even easier for schools to cease providing an education to children with disabilities in a wider range of circumstances. If these efforts had been successful, schools would have been given the opportunity to stop educating some students indefinitely without having to comply with any of the current due-process protections designed to ensure the schools' fairness and accountability.

Although the proposed amendments ultimately failed after intense opposition from parent and disability advocates, congressional supporters of IDEA, and the Administration, it is clear that many school boards, school administrators, and others involved in education policy believe that civil rights laws for children with disabilities are interfering with the ability of schools to maintain order and educate all students effectively. Outspoken school boards and their allies have fostered a climate where children receiving special education services are being scape-goated for all that is not working in American public education. If IDEA's critics are successful at further restricting the protections for children with disabilities beyond the compromise embodied in the 1997 law, the children who will suffer most will be those with disabilities with challenging behaviors, children from low-income families, racial and ethnic minority children, children in foster care, children in the juvenile justice system, and children living in rural areas without access to legal advocacy. These children are the most vulnerable to unilateral disciplinary actions by schools because these children and their families often lack the financial resources and information to challenge unfair actions or to seek appropriate alternative educational placements. The weakening of civil rights protections in IDEA would be a tragic failure in American public policy for children and families.

Moreover, if the proposed IDEA amendments are enacted, the negative impact of this change will be compounded by the recent elimination of Supplemental Security Income benefits for over 100,000 low-income children with disabilities and their families. In a period of economic prosperity, low-income families with children with disabilities are losing ground, while much of the society moves forward. This report, which updates the progress report NCD issued in 1997, will describe significant policy developments in the last year and offer recommendations for the President and the 106th Congress.

Progress, concerns and recommendations

A. Disability demographics and disability research

1. Demographics

The National Institute on Disability and Rehabilitation Research (NIDRR) at the Department of Education has published an extensive *Chartbook on Work and Disability in the United States,* 1998. The document is available in hard copy and is also excerpted on the World Wide Web.[1] The *Chartbook* draws upon data from several sources, including the Survey of Income and Program Participation, the National Health Interview Survey, the Current Population Survey, the decennial census, and the Annual Survey of Occupational Injuries and Illnesses. As noted in the *Chartbook:*

- Approximately 32 million people, or 18.7 percent of working-age Americans, report having some level of disability. Fifteen million people, or 8.7 percent of working-age Americans, report having a severe disability.[2]
- The *Chartbook* also reports statistics on the prevalence of disability by race and ethnic origin. Within the 18- to 69-year-old-age group, the following data are reported:

Ethnic Group	% Work Limitation	% Unable to Work
Native American	17.3	10.4
Black Hispanic	15.9	13.2
Black (non-Hispanic)	14.3	10.3
White (non-Hispanic)	11.6	6.2
White Hispanic	9.5	6.3
Asian or Pacific Islander[3]	5.7	3.4

- The *Chartbook* reports that there is little difference in the percentage of working-age men and women with a work disability. Approximately 8.4 million men, or 10.1 percent of the working-age male population, have a work disability. Approximately 9 million women, or 10.4 percent of the working-age female population, have a work disability. The *Chartbook* reports the following data:

Age Group	% Males	% Females	% Total Population
16-24	4.2	4.3	4.2
25-34	6.3	6.9	6.6
35-44	9.4	9.2	9.3
45-54	13.2	13.3	13.3
55-64	23.1	23.3	23.2
TOTAL	10.1	10.4	10.2

- The *Chartbook* reports that working people with disabilities have substantially lower monthly earnings than workers with no work disability, as follows:

	Median Monthly Earnings	
	Men	Women
No Disability	$2,190	$1,470
Nonsevere Disability	$1,857	$1,200
Severe Disability	$1,262	$1,000

A 1996 *Chartbook* from NIDRR reports that 4.7 million children under age 18 have activity limitations (6.7 percent of all children).[4] The breakdown of activity limitation by age follows:

Percentage of Children, By Age, With Activity Limitations

Age in Years	< 5	5-13	14-17
Limited in Nonmajor Activity	0.7	1.9	2.4
Limited in Major Activity	1.4	5.1	4.5
Unable to do Major Activity	0.6	0.6	0.7

2. Research challenges

As the figures above demonstrate, the demographics of the disability community indicate that disability policy issues should be high priority issues for policymakers, given the size and scope of the community. As the disability community grows with the aging of the baby-boom generation and as new disabilities emerge, disability policy will affect larger and larger numbers of the U.S. population. Although the employment rate of people with disabilities has received heightened attention in recent years, the employment rate for this population is not measured on a monthly basis in a manner comparable to women, blacks, and Hispanics. As part of the work of the Presidential Task Force on Employment of Adults with Disabilities, the Bureau of Labor Statistics is working with the U.S. Bureau of the Census, NIDRR, NCD and others to develop a methodology for measuring the employment rate of people with disabilities on a more regular basis.

NCD is pleased that the federal research entities are working together to improve the timeliness and accuracy of demographic and economic information regarding children and adults with disabilities. And yet, as the demographic picture of the disability population becomes more sophisticated, there remain important challenges for the research community that transcend disability demographics. For disability data and research to meet the needs of policymakers, they must measure both the population of people with disabilities and the environments with which these individuals must interact.[5]

NCD encourages NIDRR to work with the federal research community to expand efforts to measure both the characteristics of people with disabilities and the characteristics of the environment. For example, what percentage of publicly financed town homes and single-family dwellings are visitable by people in wheelchairs? What percentage of public libraries have a text telephone available to deaf and hearing-impaired patrons? What percentage of federal agency Web sites are fully accessible for blind and visually impaired computer users? What is the average lead time required to obtain paratransit services? How many health maintenance organizations allow patients to see a specialist as their primary care physician? All of these questions have important policy implications, and they cannot be answered by looking at disability demographic information alone.

B. Civil rights

At the 1996 NCD summit in Dallas, the issue of heightened enforcement of existing civil rights laws emerged as a consistent theme within many of the working groups. Although federal enforcement efforts have picked up since 1996, a need continues for stronger, more strategic, and more visible enforcement. Following up on the 1996 concerns about enforcement, NCD has undertaken a detailed analysis of federal enforcement of four civil rights laws: the Americans with Disabilities Act, the Individuals with Disabilities Education Act, the Fair Housing Act, and the Air Carrier Access Act. These reports will be issued in the first session of the 106th Congress. In the following section and in the education, transportation, and technology sections of this report, NCD analyzes specific developments in civil rights law and policy during the period covered in this report. More detailed analyses of federal enforcement efforts will appear in the statute-specific reports NCD will issue in 1999.

1. U.S. Supreme Court speaks on ADA

The United States Supreme Court heard its first two cases interpreting ADA in the last year. In the first case, *Bragdon v. Abbott*, the Court ruled that a woman who was HIV-positive but had not yet acquired symptoms associated with AIDS was nonetheless covered under ADA's definition of disability and thereby protected against discrimination when a dentist refused to fill her cavity in his office. *NCD applauds this result and encourages the Equal Employment Opportunity Commission and the Department of Justice to issue enforcement guidance using the Supreme Court's analysis to reiterate the appropriate way for courts to analyze whether a plaintiff in an ADA case is covered by the statute's definition of "disability." This guidance, coupled with the Supreme Court's decision in Abbott, should help to redirect the trend in lower courts that has narrowed the definition of disability to the point where people with breast cancer, epilepsy, diabetes, and mild mental retardation, as well as those who test positive for HIV, have been found to be outside ADA's protection.*

In the second case, *Pennsylvania Department of Corrections v. Yeskey*, the Court ruled that Title II of ADA did apply to state-run prisons. NCD applauds this result as well. In reaction to the Yeskey decision, some in Congress introduced a bill called the State and Local Prison Relief Act, which would have amended ADA and the Rehabilitation Act to exempt state and local agencies operating prisons from the civil rights requirements of the two laws. This bill was not enacted into law in the last Congress but may return in the new Congress. *NCD encourages the President and Congress to oppose any amendments to ADA or the Rehabilitation Act that would narrow the scope of protections they provide. Rather than mounting legal challenges to the constitutionality of Title II of ADA, as many states have attempted with limited success, the newly elected and incumbent governors and attorneys general at the state level should be expected to embrace the civil rights requirements of ADA and seek cost-effective ways to bring the instruments of state and local government into compliance.*

Although the Supreme Court decisions in Bragdon and Yeskey should help to correct some of the disturbing trends in federal court decisions under ADA, federal judges still need to develop greater understanding of the principles of ADA and other disability civil rights laws. This can be accomplished through continuing education programs for the bench. In addition, the President and Congress need to work together to find, appoint, and confirm qualified lawyers and judges with disabilities and with a good understanding of the legal and philosophical underpinnings of the disability civil rights movement to the federal bench.

2. Hate crimes

Congress acted this past year on the civil rights issue of hate crimes. On November 13, 1997, a Hate Crimes bill was introduced that would have increased the penalty for people convicted of hate crimes against people with disabilities. This bill did not ultimately pass, but another bill was enacted that requires the collection of data on the commission of hate crimes against people with disabilities. The data called for in the new law will make it easier to establish the need for legislation similar to the bill introduced in November 1997 and will help protect any such legislation from a constitutional challenge. *NCD commends Congress and the President for recognizing the need for the collection of data on hate crimes against people with disabilities and encourages the 106th Congress and the President to revisit this issue by passing a law that includes a stronger penalty and appropriate rehabilitation for people convicted of committing such crimes.*

3. Civil rights enforcement

a. U.S. Equal Employment Opportunity Commission (EEOC)
In part as a result of activities and recommendations associated with PIR, Congress approved a $37 million increase in the EEOC budget. This increase, the first significant budget increase for EEOC since it received the added enforcement responsibility of ADA, is an important first step toward giving EEOC the resources to investigate claims in a timely manner and to provide badly needed outreach and technical assistance to its many stakeholders. *NCD commends Congress and the President for increasing EEOC's appropriations and encourages EEOC to use the increase to enhance customer service in the field and to train investigators on the quickly developing case law under ADA.*
b. Department of Housing and Urban Development
Also as part of PIR, the President proposed and Congress approved a significant expansion in the Department of Housing and Urban Development's (HUD's) fair housing enforcement budget for Fiscal

Year (FY) 1999. The approved budget for fair housing programs was $40 million, up from $30 million in FY 1998. *NCD commends the President and Congress for recognizing the need to expand fair housing enforcement. NCD recommends that HUD use the increase in appropriations for fair housing to expand its enforcement of the Fair Housing Act and section 504 of the Rehabilitation Act on behalf of people with disabilities. To the extent that HUD will be doubling enforcement efforts under the Fair Housing Act, for example, NCD recommends that HUD's efforts under section 504 also be doubled.*

In early summer 1998, the Fair Housing and Equal Opportunity (FHEO) division at HUD amended its standard compliance review procedure to include, for the first time, a review for section 504 compliance as part of any fair housing compliance assessment. *NCD commends HUD for recognizing the need to integrate section 504 compliance monitoring within its generic fair housing compliance activities.*

In early 1998, HUD began a large-scale inspection effort, whereby it is systematically reviewing the physical plants of HUD-financed projects to assess compliance with many different safety and conservation standards. As part of this effort, HUD inspectors are assessing compliance with accessibility laws and regulations, such as section 504 of the Rehabilitation Act. *NCD commends HUD for doing this and encourages HUD to make the accessibility results public.*

In summer 1998, HUD's division of Policy Development and Research, along with FHEO, contracted with a private research firm to conduct a national survey of all newly constructed multifamily housing (with four or more contiguous units) built since March 1991 (the effective date of the Fair Housing Act's new construction guidelines). This survey will gather data to provide statistically reliable information on the numbers, types and locations of buildings that do and do not comply with the Fair Housing Act. *NCD commends HUD for recognizing the need for comprehensive information in this area and encourages HUD to make the results of this survey public.*

In April 1998, HUD published a Fair Housing Guidelines Design Manual intended to further illustrate ways for buildings to comply with the new construction requirements of the Fair Housing Act. Some developers have pointed to the 1998 issuance of this document to argue that they should not be held liable for failing to comply with the Fair Housing Act's accessibility requirements for buildings that were built after the 1991 effective date of the law but before the 1998 guidelines. *NCD commends HUD for issuing these important guidelines and strongly encourages HUD to resist any efforts to eliminate liability for developers who built multifamily units between 1991 and the April 1998 publication of the Fair Housing Guidelines Design Manual.*

c. Department of Justice

Along with the EEOC and HUD increases, Congress approved an increase of a little more than $1 million for the Department of Justice's

(DOJ's) Civil Rights Division to increase enforcement and mediation activities under ADA. *NCD commends Congress and the President for increasing the appropriation for ADA enforcement at DOJ. It encourages DOJ to expand its efforts to coordinate ADA enforcement across all the agencies, particularly in the areas of most integrated setting requirements under Title II; technology access issues under Titles II and III; and compliance by elementary, secondary, and postsecondary schools under Title II.*

4. Civil rights backlash

The backlash against civil rights for people with disabilities continued to show its face in the last year. Commentators and pundits continue to complain about the "wrong people" benefitting from ADA and about the extraordinary costs being incurred by employers, particularly for litigation. Critics argue that ADA is a failure because the employment rate for people with disabilities has not increased significantly since the law's passage and because of the perception that the law is vague and difficult to interpret with certainty. None of these arguments withstand close scrutiny, yet they resurface consistently.

NCD encourages ADA enforcement agencies like EEOC, DOJ, and DOT to recognize that part of their mission as enforcement agencies must be to correct misperceptions or inaccuracies about ADA that only serve to feed the backlash. When an article is published that clearly misconstrues ADA, it is essential that the agency in the best position to respond does so in a timely and effective manner. If not, myths are allowed to disguise themselves as facts, and the environment for successful enforcement is compromised.

5. Access to the electoral process

The right to vote is one of the most fundamental civil and human rights in a democracy. Yet, many people with disabilities are not able to exercise this right fully because local elections are not accessible to them. In 1984, Congress attempted to resolve this problem by enacting the Voting Accessibility for the Elderly and Handicapped Act (VAA). Although this law was an important first step in recognizing and addressing voting access issues, it has not eliminated the widespread problems people with disabilities encounter with polling places and polling methods (e.g. voting booths and ballots). The law includes no effective remedy for individuals who are harmed by inaccessible polling places and fails to establish any national standard for accessibility.

Notwithstanding the weaknesses of VAA, some jurisdictions have been more proactive than others in ensuring access for voters with disabilities. In Rhode Island, for example, the state Board of Elections worked with the Governor's Commission on Disabilities to make 94 percent of the state's polling places accessible in time for the September 1998 primary elections. State officials also made provisions for assistance to individuals with disabilities who live in the inaccessible polling place neighborhoods.

NCD encourages the President and Congress to recognize that the ability of a person with a disability to vote should not depend on the goodwill of the state election agency but instead should be guaranteed as a federally protected civil right with real consequences when the right is violated. Accordingly, NCD encourages the President and Congress to enact legislation that would amend VAA to recognize the right of all individuals to vote independently; guarantee accessibility to all stages of the electoral process (from voter registration to election day procedures); require the Architectural and Transportation Barriers Compliance Board ("Access Board") to establish standards for the accessibility of polling places, polling methods, and registration materials; strengthen the law's enforcement mechanisms to ensure private individuals are able to enforce their rights; and require regular and meaningful monitoring of access to elections for people with disabilities by the Federal Election Commission or other appropriate entity.

6. Wilderness accessibility

Section 507(a) of ADA required that NCD identify important issues relevant to wilderness accessibility for people with disabilities. On December 1, 1992, NCD issued a report entitled *Wilderness Accessibility for People with Disabilities*, which included recommendations developed after a hearing and preliminary study of the issue. A key recommendation in the report was that the federal agencies responsible for wilderness management should better coordinate their policies and management practices regarding disability access and make them consistent with the requirements of federal nondiscrimination laws. In October 1997, a memorandum of understanding was signed by the federal wilderness management agencies and a nonprofit organization called Wilderness Inquiry, Inc. (WI), to coordinate their policies to "establish a general framework of cooperation between the agencies and WI for increased opportunities for people of all abilities to use and enjoy the programs, facilities, and activities of the agencies." In the last days of the 105th Congress, related legislation was passed that requires the secretary of agriculture and the secretary of the interior to conduct a comprehensive study to improve the access for persons with disabilities to outdoor recreational opportunities (such as fishing, hunting, trapping, wildlife viewing, hiking, boating, and camping) made available to the public on the federal lands in the National Forest System, the National Park System, the National Wildlife Refuge System, and the Bureau of Land Management.

C. Education

1. Omnibus fiscal year 1999 budget bill

The final budget bill signed by the President included $1.2 billion for the first year of the President's initiative to hire 100,000 new teachers to reduce class size in the early grades to a national average of 18. This initiative is designed to help schools recruit high quality teachers and to insure that students receive more individual attention, a solid foundation in the basics, and greater discipline in the classroom. *NCD commends the President and Congress for providing funding to hire new teachers and reduce class size. NCD encourages the President and the Department of Education (DOE) to work to ensure that the new teachers have the proper training to meet the special needs of children with disabilities in mainstream classrooms. Moreover, NCD encourages the President and Congress to continue to work together to fund the hiring of additional new teachers in the upcoming FY 2000 budget discussions. Finally, NCD encourages the DOE to work to ensure that the new teachers hired as a result of the new funding represent a diverse cross-section of the communities they will serve, including people with disabilities. Teachers with disabilities, like teachers from other disenfranchised groups, represent important role models and can change school cultures with their example and their presence.*

The final budget bill also included new funding for after-school programs, child literacy, college mentoring for middle school children, education technology, child care quality, teacher recruitment, Head Start, charter schools, a Hispanic education initiative, Pell grants, and summer jobs. *NCD commends the President and Congress for investing in expanding programs aimed at children and youth. NCD strongly encourages the administering agencies for these new funds to ensure that the recipients of the funds take steps to include children and youth with disabilities in their activities. For example, the education technology funding should be spent on technology that is accessible for all students, including students with visual, hearing, learning and mobility impairments. Likewise, recipients of new charter school funding should be required to demonstrate their ability to serve students with a range of disabilities in mainstream settings.*

2. School modernization

Having failed in the final days of Congress to prevail in his push for school-construction funding, President Clinton likely will seek again to modernize public schools around the country by using tax credits to leverage nearly $22 billion in bonds to build and renovate schools. *NCD strongly supports the President's initiative to modernize our schools. It encourages the President and Congress to work together to find the funds to support this initiative, and then to ensure that the newly built or renovated schools are models of universal design so that all students, teachers, and parents will be able to participate fully in all aspects of the schools of the future.*

3. IDEA proposals

Less than five months after the IDEA Amendments of 1997 (IDEA 1997) were signed into law on June 4, 1997, DOE issued a Notice of Proposed Rulemaking (NPRM) inviting public comment on the proposed regulations by January 20, 1998. As of October 31, 1998, no final regulations had been issued. An achievement of bipartisan compromise, the enactment of IDEA 1997 followed months of intense political struggle to block reauthorization. As noted in the introduction to this report, the struggle resurfaced this year in a flurry of measures in the House and Senate designed to block or to erode key provisions of the law. These amendments, summarized later, have sought to limit the civil rights protections of IDEA in the name of greater flexibility for schools.

Several amendments proposed changes affecting due-process protections in the administration of school discipline procedures. Current law allows removal of students to an interim alternative educational setting (IAES) for up to 45 days at a time only when they bring a weapon to school, commit a drug-related offense at school, or have been found by an independent hearing officer to be substantially likely to injure themselves or others. One amendment, referenced in the Introduction, proposed to allow schools to remove unilaterally students who intentionally exhibit violent behavior that has, or could have, resulted in injury to themselves or others, even if the behavior was a manifestation of the disability. The amendment would have replaced objective decisionmaking by an impartial and independent hearing officer with unilateral fact-finding and decisionmaking by the school. Finally, this amendment proposed to delete the 45-day limit on exclusion of students from their regular classroom, which would eliminate protection against indefinite removal without review. A more extreme variation on this amendment would have provided that, notwithstanding IDEA, state and local educational agencies could establish and implement uniform discipline policies applying to all children within their jurisdictions. School personnel would be permitted unilaterally to expel children with disabilities whose behavior was disruptive, even if related to their disability, regardless of any IDEA provision.

A second provision targeted for amendment was the right to educational services for youth with disabilities incarcerated as adults. The proposed amendment in this area would have made it impossible for DOE to reduce or withhold payments from states for failure to provide special education and related services to these children after age 18. As proposed, this provision would have effectively eliminated access to appropriate educational services by young prisoners in many states.

Finally, IDEA provides for the payment of attorneys' fees to parents who are prevailing parties in actions or proceedings brought under section 615 of the Act. Language imbedded in the House District of Columbia appropriations bill would have: 1) eliminated attorneys' fees for administrative hearings, which make up the bulk of special education cases, and 2) limited attorney compensation to $50/hour for cases filed in court, with a cap of $1,300 per case.

Each of these amendments directly challenged the core premises of IDEA: that each child with a disability has the right to a free appropriate public education (FAPE) in the least restrictive environment consistent with that goal, has due process protections against unilateral actions by the school, and has access to an effective remedy when schools fail to comply with their obligations. After a fierce battle, the discipline amendments were dropped in exchange for a nine-month study of the effect of federal special education protections on the ability of schools to maintain discipline. This study will be conducted by the U.S. General Accounting Office. All of the other amendments were dropped, except the cap on attorneys' fees in the District of Columbia, which remained in the final appropriations bill approved by Congress. Many fear that the D.C. measure is the trial balloon for a broader attempt to cap attorneys' fees, which would make it even less likely that a family with a child with a disability would be able to assert their legal rights in court.

Advocates devoted significant energy and resources this year to opposing these attempts to weaken the law and encouraging DOE to strengthen the proposed regulations and issue the final regulations as quickly as possible. While the NPRM mirrors or strengthens the provisions of IDEA 1997 for the most part, significant weak areas remain. Among them are temporary suspension of educational services following short-term removal from the classroom, lack of specific timelines for completing important actions, unclear requirements concerning the notification and inclusion of parents in key meetings and decisions, and only partial inclusion of requirements for the early intervention program (Part C). After receiving thousands of comments on the NPRM, DOE moved the release date for the final regulation from late spring to December 1998.

NCD recommends that the DOE promptly issue the final regulations implementing IDEA 1997. The regulations will serve as both a safeguard and guidance to the educational system at state and local levels. NCD strongly encourages local jurisdictions to use the federal regulation as a model in developing their own guidelines for implementing IDEA and incorporating best practices drawing on their local successes.

Along with opposition in Congress and concomitant delays at DOE, IDEA continues to be met with noncompliance and outright opposition at the state and local level. Feedback from national parent networks indicates that opposition to IDEA and the protections it affords arise from five core perceptions: (1) students with disabilities require more than their fair share of educational resources, which makes it more difficult for schools to educate the rest of their students; (2) the unfettered ability of schools to exclude children with challenging behaviors is necessary to ensure school safety; (3) IDEA paperwork requirements (i.e., the Individual Education Plan [IEP]) divert resources from educating children; (4) IDEA imposes requirements that take away control from state and local education agencies, and (5) schools do not want to deal with difficult children in mainstream settings.

Parents around the country report strong resistance on the part of school personnel and administrators to providing appropriate services for their children. At the same time, powerful education associations lobby to give local school personnel authority to cease education for students with disabilities without due process. In many school districts, parents must continually fight for services required by IDEA, which indicates that noncompliance may be widespread and largely unchallenged.

NCD recommends that DOE and DOJ recognize and correct the inadequacy of current federal compliance monitoring activity. School systems that fail to provide services required under IDEA are compromising the futures of children with disabilities. Federal authorities must develop more effective monitoring mechanisms to identify and challenge failures to comply. School systems found not in compliance must be held accountable for correcting deficiencies within specified time frames or face sanctions. Where the will to fully implement IDEA is lacking, sanctions must be applied in combination with positive incentives to change resistance to definitive action.

Providing all children access to FAPE requires many changes to our existing educational systems. Rather than expecting all children to achieve on the same terms, FAPE requires collaboration between parents and school personnel in accommodating the needs of individual children. It requires a systematic approach to supporting each child's individual ability and excellence, which means an alternative approach to the allocation of educational resources. It requires acquiring and integrating assistive technologies into the classroom that have not been available previously. It requires drawing on expertise from a variety of sources, rather than expecting one educator to address all the needs of a child with a disability. Implementing IDEA requires a commitment to change, as well as an increase and a reallocation of resources at the national, state, and local levels.

Federal policy must support solutions aimed at directing resources toward creating safe and inclusive educational environments; thorough, yet manageable, information management systems; and collaboration between parents and state and local school personnel in meeting the educational needs of all students.

NCD recommends that the President and Congress make good on the 1975 commitment to allocate to the states 40 percent of the funding needed to implement IDEA. This year Congress approved funding at 12 percent, which is the highest level yet, but still far short of what is needed. Also, in light of the fact that the federal government has increased its share of funding for IDEA by approximately $1.5 billion over the last three years, NCD encourages the DOE to assess what local schools have been able to accomplish with these additional funds. Are teachers receiving better training in ways to meet the needs of children with disabilities? Have early intervention programs been expanded for infants and toddlers with disabilities? Are funds being used to empower parents of children with disabilities by providing parent training and information about IDEA?

NCD recommends that state education agencies assist local school systems in organizing, simplifying and standardizing IDEA's information requirements to make compliance easier and to develop meaningful data for measuring results.

Finally, NCD urges educators across the country to view IDEA as a national commitment to educating all children, regardless of their circumstances, and to accept the challenge of reshaping their local education systems to be responsive to the needs of individual students. Developing collaborative models for interaction between parents, school personnel, and students will be a key strategy in creating this responsiveness and removing the barriers to FAPE for all students with disabilities.

4. Charter public schools

The Administration has been generally supportive of charter public schools as a laboratory for innovation in American public education. As previously noted, the final budget bill included increased federal funding for public charter schools. The Administration and many in Congress have indicated a desire to see charter schools continue to grow in number with federal support.

NCD is concerned that public charter schools are being created in some jurisdictions without actually ensuring that the teachers and administrators are prepared to comply with IDEA, ADA and section 504 of the Rehabilitation Act when children with disabilities seek to enroll. NCD encourages DOE to provide technical assistance, oversight, monitoring, and enforcement to the growing number of charter schools in best practices for educating students with disabilities.

5. Elementary and Secondary Education Act

One of the items on the agenda for the 106th Congress will be the reauthorization of the Elementary and Secondary Education Act (ESEA), an important law that sets out federal education policy for all students, particularly students from low-income families. ESEA currently requires states to set high standards for all students, to create quality assessments that measure how well students are meeting those standards, and to create an accountability system for schools to ensure that schools are making progress toward preparing students to meet the standards. Under ESEA, schools must provide an enriched and accelerated curriculum, effective instructional methods, high-quality professional staff, high-quality professional development, and timely and effective individual assistance for students who are struggling to meet standards. Schools must meet all of these elements in a program developed in partnership with parents.

NCD encourages the President and Congress to take advantage of the opportunity provided by the ESEA reauthorization to address the need for mainstream education policy to integrate the needs of students with disabilities and students from low-income families so that the educational outcomes of all students may be improved. For example, NCD encourages the President and Congress to use the reauthorization to ensure that students with disabilities are meaningfully included in standards-based reform and expected to meet high standards, with appropriate accommodations; to expand parent training and information efforts by building upon and promoting linkages with community-based parent training and information centers funded under IDEA, so that all parents can work together to promote high-quality programming that meets the individual needs of all students; and to improve teacher training and professional development to better meet the diverse needs of students in mainstream settings.

6. Education of the Deaf Amendments of 1998

As part of the Higher Education Amendments of 1998 passed by Congress and signed by the President, the Education of the Deaf Act was amended to require elementary and secondary programs to comply with certain require-ments of IDEA, among other things. The legislation also requires the secre-tary of education to study and report to Congress on the education of the deaf to identify those education-related factors in the lives of deaf individuals that result in barriers to successful postsecondary education experiences and employment, or contribute to successful postsecondary education and employment experiences. *NCD commends the President and Congress for rec-ognizing the importance of conducting a thorough study of the factors in public education of deaf students that impede or promote their success after secondary school, and encourages the secretary of education to act promptly to complete the study and report.*

D. Health care

1. Protections in managed care

Like the education system, the health care system is an essential infrastruc-ture that can either facilitate functional ability and choice for people with disabilities or make it difficult for people with disabilities to achieve their goals. With the vast majority of people in private insurance and a growing percentage of the Medicaid population enrolled in managed care, people with disabilities have a strong stake in the efforts to create rights for patients in managed care systems. In the last year, the President and many in Con-gress worked to pass a "patient's bill of rights," which would include patient protections such as assuring access to specialists; creating strong emergency room protections; continuity of care provisions to prevent abrupt changes in treatment; a fair, timely, and independent appeals process for patient grievances; and enforcement provisions to make these rights real. *NCD strongly encourages the President and the 106th Congress to overcome partisan differences and work together to forge a strong, enforceable bill that will give patients with disabilities and their families sufficient protections to ensure that they have access to the quality health care they need. In addition, NCD recommends that the President and Congress work together to address the unique issues managed care has created in medical rehabilitation, where people with disabilities are being forced to leave rehabilitation hospitals prematurely and are not receiving the range of necessary services and supports that medical rehabilitation professionals provided before the growth of managed care.*

2. Medicare reform

Another big item on the health care agenda is the future of the Medicare program. Much like the debate on Social Security solvency, the discussions around the future of Medicare have largely taken place with little or no involvement by people with disabilities. Despite the fact that many working-age people with disabilities rely on Medicare and the health care provided along with their SSDI benefits, this population has been virtually ignored in the Medicare discussions to date. *NCD encourages the President, Congress, and the Bipartisan Commission on the Future of Medicare to involve people with dis-*

abilities and their advocates in the discussions about what should happen with the Medicare program. At a minimum, the commission should reach out to working-age Medicare enrollees with disabilities to obtain their input on how the program might better meet their needs. As it stands currently, Medicare is much more effective for elderly enrollees than it is for working-age people with disabilities because it is structured with the needs of the elderly in mind. To the extent that changes are being considered, NCD encourages the President and Congress to consider making the scope of coverage under Medicare more in line with the kinds of services and supports needed by working-age people with disabilities.

3. Medicaid buy-in

In 1997, NCD reported on the provision in the Balanced Budget Act of that year that created an optional program whereby states could allow people with disabilities who were earning up to 250 percent of poverty to purchase Medicaid coverage. This past year, HHS Secretary Donna Shalala personally wrote to every state to encourage implementation of this provision. To date, NCD is aware of only one state, Oregon, that has taken advantage of this option. Oregon amended its state Medicaid plan, with approval from HCFA, and is in the process of writing its administrative rules and implementation procedures. The Oregon program will be similar to section 1619(b) but offers Medicaid to working individuals who have unearned income, higher income levels, and others. The program will let individuals go to work and get and keep Medicaid, even if their income exceeds $40,000. *NCD commends Oregon for being the first state in the nation to take advantage of the 1997 Balanced Budget Act provision and encourages other states to follow Oregon's lead and expand health care options available to their populations of people with disabilities when they are working.*

4. Assisted suicide

On another front, this year witnessed an attempt in Michigan to follow Oregon's lead in legalizing physician-assisted suicide. Although it acknowledges differences of opinion in the disability community on this topic, NCD opposes legalization of physician-assisted suicide because of the real danger that this practice, if made legal, will be used in a discriminatory manner against individuals with disabilities. As of October 31, voters in Dr. Jack Kevorkian's home state were poised to reject a measure that would have made Michigan the second state with legalized physician-assisted suicide.

The measure, known locally as Proposal B, was headed for defeat according to the polls, which in weeks before the election showed support eroding under a multi-million-dollar advertising campaign by well-funded opponents, including the Michigan State Medical Society, the Roman Catholic Church and Right to Life of Michigan. Disability rights groups, particularly Not Dead Yet, also were vocal in their opposition to the measure.

Opposition also came from Kevorkian, who says he has attended more than 120 deaths but considered Proposal B too restrictive and regulatory. He called the proposal "crazy."

The measure would have allowed doctors in some cases to prescribe a lethal dose of medication for terminally ill patients wishing to kill themselves. It got on the ballot through an effort by Merian's Friends, a group named after a woman who died with Kevorkian's involvement.

NCD commends the voters in Michigan for recognizing the problems inherent with the legalization of physician-assisted suicide, and encourages the President and Congress to speak out against this dangerous and unnecessary expansion of the physician's role. Health care should be about healing, not killing.[6]

Another important development in this area occurred in Congress. In response to the failure of DOJ to take action against physicians prescribing lethal drugs under federal controlled substances laws, some in Congress introduced the Lethal Drug Abuse Prevention Act of 1998. Although the bill was not enacted, it did receive a hearing before the Constitution Subcommittee of the House Judiciary Committee. Diane Coleman from the disability rights group Not Dead Yet testified at the hearing. *NCD commends the Constitution Subcommittee for recognizing the importance of including a disability rights perspective in discussions about assisted suicide, and NCD encourages the President to work with Congress to craft a federal law that will protect the human rights of people with disabilities and restrain the ability of physicians to prescribe lethal drugs.*

E. Long-term services and supports for individuals and families

A necessary corollary to an effective acute care system is an affordable system for long-term services and supports for individuals and families. The biggest problem with the current system from the perspective of children and adults with disabilities and their families is the lack of real choices it offers people in need of long-term supports. Because of the institutional bias in the Medicaid statute, where nursing home care is mandatory in every state but home- and community-based care is optional, approximately 80 percent of the funding for long-term services and supports goes to services in institutions. This continues to occur notwithstanding the fact that the vast majority of people with disabilities of all ages and their families would prefer that the services be delivered in home- and community-based settings.

1. Federal legislative efforts

As mentioned in the Introduction to this report, in March 1998, the House subcommittee with jurisdiction over Medicaid held a hearing on MiCASA, which was developed with the disability rights group ADAPT and attracted many sponsors on both sides of the aisle. Approximately 50 national disability and aging groups have indicated their support of MiCASA. At the hearing, Speaker Newt Gingrich and Minority Leader Richard Gephardt both testified eloquently about the need for legislation that would enable people with disabilities to choose to live outside of nursing homes and other institutional settings, and many witnesses presented compelling testimony about the institutional bias in the current system and the failure of federal and state policy to honor the "most integrated setting" goals articulated in ADA for delivery of state and local services. Nonetheless, very little happened in the last Congress that moved the ball forward on national legislation to remove the institutional bias in the Medicaid system. Senator Russell Feingold's bill, modeled on the long-term care provisions of President Clinton's Health Security Act, likewise received little attention from the Finance Committee in the Senate, which is the committee of jurisdiction. *NCD encourages the 106th Congress to move beyond rhetoric and implement a strategy for dramatically expanding consumer choice in long-term care. As the population ages, the crisis currently being felt among many seniors and people with disabilities who require assistance with activities of daily living will only become more widespread.*

2. Administration efforts

On a more positive note, the Administration took steps in the last year to call attention to ADA's requirement that home- and community-based services, like other government-funded services, be delivered in the "most integrated setting" appropriate so that people with disabilities do not receive services in segregated settings unnecessarily. As Attorney General Janet Reno said before the National Council on Independent Living in May,

> We believe that states have an obligation to provide services to people with disabilities in the most integrated setting appropriate to their needs. And we have used the law to fight for this. Many individuals with disabilities are being placed in nursing homes or other institutional settings even when they don't really need to be there.

On a similar note, Sally Richardson, who directs the Medicaid program for HCFA, issued a directive to state Medicaid directors in conjunction with the ADA anniversary at the end of July that pointed out ADA's requirement that state and local services be delivered in the most integrated setting appropriate to the service. *NCD commends the President; Secretary Shalala; Nancy-Ann Min DeParle, administrator of HCFA; Sally Richardson, director of the Center for Medicaid and State Operations at HCFA; and Robert Williams, deputy assistant secretary for disability and long-term care policy at HHS, for working together to issue the directive to Medicaid directors regarding ADA's implications in the area of Medicaid services. NCD also encourages HCFA to stand firm behind its letter and resist state efforts to read the letter in a manner that enables them to deliver services in the same manner to which they have grown accustomed. NCD encourages HHS to provide technical assistance to states on how to comply with the most integrated setting requirement in the Medicaid program. At the same time, NCD encourages the Administration to fund an initiative as part of its FY 2000 budget that will enable states to transition from a system that focuses on institutions to one that focuses on home- and community-based services.*

3. Family support

Like adults with disabilities, many families of children with disabilities have advocated for long-term services and supports for their children and for family caregivers to enable families to care for their children at home and outside of institutions. In 1994, Congress created a new part in the Individuals with Disabilities Education Act which authorized HHS to fund state efforts to promote systems change at the state level that would enhance services and supports for families of children with disabilities. This authorization effectively expired on October 1, 1998, without being reauthorized. However, President Clinton inserted and Congress approved a line item in the FY 1999 budget that allocated $4 million for family support. These funds will be used to support 17 competitive grants to conduct projects of national significance in the area of family support.

Accordingly, for the first time, the President and Congress have recognized the need to fund a family support program for families of children with disabilities. *NCD commends the President and Congress for allocating funds to support systems change at the state level that will enhance the ability of families to care for their children at home and outside of institutions. At the same time, NCD encourages the President and Congress to reauthorize in statute an ongoing family support program administered by HHS, possibly as part of the reauthorization of the Developmental Disabilities Assistance and Bill of Rights Act.*

4. Child care

In the omnibus budget bill approved at the end of the 105th Congress, the Child Care and Development Block Grant (CCDBG) received $172 million specifically to promote quality in the delivery of child care services. This money has been used in the past and can be used in the future for technical assistance activities to support best practices in the area of inclusion of children with disabilities in mainstream child care programs. In addition, Congress and the President supplemented the budget for after-school care by $140 million. This money may be used to expand the availability of after-school programs for all children, including children with disabilities. *NCD commends the President and Congress for making available funds to improve child care options for children with disabilities and their families. NCD encourages HHS and DOE to work with the state and local governments to ensure that children with disabilities are integrated into the child care and after-school care networks developed with the new funding. Also, in light of the fact that 24 states currently have waiting lists for children to get into quality child care programs, NCD encourages the President and the 106th Congress to continue to expand the federal commitment to ensure that all children have access to quality, affordable, accessible child care.*

F. Immigrants, racial and ethnic minorities with disabilities

NCD has worked for many years to address the unique needs of minorities with disabilities in our policy work. Recently, NCD has hosted roundtable discussions and hearings in Atlanta, New Orleans, and San Francisco on the issues facing people with disabilities from minority and rural communities from different sections of the country. On October 1, 1998, NCD released a report capturing input from the January 1998 hearing in New Orleans focused on children and youth with disabilities and their families from minority and rural communities in Louisiana.[7] The report included suggestions and recommendations on a range of issues, including education, vocational rehabilitation, juvenile justice, access to medical services, independent living, family and individual support, and community participation. Early in 1999, NCD will issue a report that captures input from its hearing in San Francisco in August 1998. NCD is eager to work with the President and Congress to redouble federal efforts to tailor federal policies and programs so they appropriately address the unique issues facing people with disabilities from minority racial and ethnic communities.

1. President's Initiative on Race

Over the past year PIR has sponsored research and discussions around the country to facilitate education and cooperation on race issues in America. In September, the PIR Advisory Board presented to President Clinton its final report, which details the activities undertaken and the policy recommendations developed to reduce social and economic division by race. Although minimal attention was given to race issues related to disability (including co-sponsorship with NCD of an August discussion involving community leaders in San Francisco), overall the effort to hear from and comment on the unique issues facing minorities with disabilities has been inadequate, and significant opportunities have been missed. *NCD hopes that the President will seek to remedy the situation in his expected report to the American people based on this initiative.*

Research studies, including the National Health Interview Survey statistics previously cited, consistently show that people from diverse cultural communities experience higher rates of disability as a result of living conditions such as poorer health care coverage, greater exposure to violent crimes, nutrition issues, and increased presence of environmental pollutants. The problems resulting from higher rates of disability are compounded by weaker disability support systems, including education and employment settings that are less informed and equipped to address accessibility needs of people with disabilities. Accordingly, it is in the interest of racial and ethnic minorities, at least as much as others, to advocate public policies and resources that promote the personal independence, social integration, and economic empowerment of Americans with disabilities.

In addition to the problems faced by people with disabilities of all races, some particularly affect people who are members of racial and ethnic minority groups. Navigating the immigration and naturalization process, for example, can be harder when one has a disability that affects one's ability to learn English through standard instructional methods, affects one's capability to give fingerprints (a man without fingers has had his naturalization delayed for years because of this problem), or affects one's capacity to give the oath of allegiance. Despite the fact that civil rights laws protect immigrants with disabilities against rigid application of citizenship requirements, NCD has heard numerous individual reports of the Immigration and Naturalization Service's refusal to make accommodations. Another example is that some cultures have not yet developed language about disability that makes it acceptable to self-identify, request, and receive government interventions such as civil rights enforcement and rehabilitation services. Through dialogues and research in conjunction with the disability community, PIR could have advanced understanding in these areas and helped to encourage more enabling policies and practices for minorities with disabilities.

NCD does commend PIR for recognizing in its report a pattern at the local level of giving special education labels to children with disabilities from minority backgrounds, which results in many of them being unnecessarily stigmatized and separated from mainstream education settings. Regulations to be issued by DOE implementing the IDEA Amendments of 1997 can and should correct this practice. NCD also praises the President's action in July to direct key federal civil rights agencies to increase their outreach and implementation efforts in diverse cultural communities. *NCD urges federal civil rights enforcement agencies to work together to develop culturally competent models for outreach and training on federal civil rights laws and procedures in minority racial and ethnic communities.*

2. Health-related funding in minority communities

In the final budget bill that passed at the end of the 105th Congress, $150 million was included to address HIV/AIDS issues in minority communities. This investment will be used to improve prevention efforts in high-risk communities and expand access to cutting-edge HIV therapies and other treatment needed for HIV/AIDS. In addition, Congress approved the Administration's request to fund grants for communities to develop new strategies to address disparities in prevalence of diseases between minority and white populations. Among African Americans under the age of 65, for example, the rate of heart disease is twice the rate among whites in that age group. As another example, Native Americans have an incidence of diabetes nearly three times the national average. As part of the President's initiative to eliminate racial health disparities, Congress also approved increases in other public health programs, such as heart disease and diabetes prevention at the Centers for Disease Control, that have proven effective in attacking these disparities. *NCD commends the President and Congress for recognizing the need to pay particular attention to disability issues in minority communities. As the President and Congress continue to build on these first steps, NCD encourages them to address the dramatic disparities in labor force participation between minorities with disabilities and others.*

F. Social Security work incentives and Social Security solvency

1. Work incentives

As mentioned in the Introduction, this Congress saw significant progress toward making it easier for people receiving Social Security disability benefits to go back to work, but ultimately no bill was passed by both houses of Congress. On September 24, 1997, NCD presented the President and Congress with a list of action proposals to remove barriers to work.[8] The proposals, which were developed after broad consultation with people with disabilities, their families, advocates, and policy experts around the country, included actions that would "make work pay" by providing medical coverage for workers with disabilities, replacing the SSDI income cliff with gradual benefit reductions, ensuring that people would not lose eligibility solely because they work, compensating for disability-related work incentives, and other items. The NCD recommendations also supported the creation of a ticket or voucher program that would enable SSI recipients and SSDI beneficiaries to select and buy services leading to employment and the creation of a financial reimbursement mechanism for employers who encounter costs for certain extraordinary accommodations.

On June 4, 1998, the House voted 410-1 to pass the Ticket to Work and Self-Sufficiency Act. This bill would have instituted a ticket program similar to the NCD proposal designed to increase consumer choice in vocational rehabilitation. It also would have authorized a demonstration project in which a select group of beneficiaries would have lost cash benefits at a rate of one dollar for every two dollars they earned over an amount to be determined by the commissioner of Social Security. The House bill did not include the national two-for-one proposal espoused by NCD because that proposal had received a large score from Congressional Budget Office and the actuaries at SSA, both of which were concerned about people being induced by that benefit to come onto the rolls.

The Work Incentives Improvements Act in the Senate included a ticket component similar to NCD's and the House bill and included a demonstration program for the two-for-one similar to the House bill. In addition, it included significant health care protections for SSI and SSDI beneficiaries that would have enabled them to keep their health care when they returned to work. Another important component of the Senate bill was the definition of personal assistance services that would have been part of the health coverage — a definition that included readers and personal assistance with transportation to and from work. Finally, both the Senate and House bills included provisions that would have prevented the Social Security Administration from punishing people who try to work by instituting a continuing disability review.

An important consensus that emerged as the 105th Congress drew to a close was the realization that the disability community was not interested in a work incentives bill that did not include a significant health care protection for people trying to leave the Social Security rolls. Because the health care component was significantly more costly than the other components of the legislation, it was necessarily the most difficult to achieve. *NCD encourages the President, commissioner of Social Security, and Congress to build on the progress made last year and pass a work incentives bill that includes basic access to health care and expanded choice in rehabilitation providers for consumers similar to the Work Incentives Improvements Act. NCD encourages the Administration and Congress to fund the health care components of the bill at a level that will make them sufficiently attractive for states to choose to participate.*

2. Social Security Solvency

As mentioned in the Introduction, people with disabilities have not played a large or visible role in discussions about the solvency of the Social Security Trust Fund to date. Accordingly, many Americans have a perception that Social Security is only for people who have retired, and the debate about solvency has centered almost exclusively on Social Security retirement. Yet, the reform efforts that will play out in the 106th Congress will have a dramatic impact on the people with disabilities who depend on SSDI benefits to survive. More than one-third of all Social Security benefits are paid to nonretirees: people with disabilities, children, and widowed spouses. For the average wage earner with a family, Social Security insurance benefits are equivalent to a $300,000 life insurance policy or a $200,000 disability insurance policy.

As the debate moves forward, NCD encourages the President and Congress to:

- *Ensure the meaningful inclusion of people with disabilities and their families in discussions about the projected shortfall of the Trust Fund;*
- *Preserve the guarantees inherent in the disability insurance program and the protections for survivors and dependents in the Old Age, Survivors, and Disability Insurance programs of Title II of the Social Security Act;*
- *Protect the integrity of the benefits provided so that they are at a reasonable level for support and protect the value of the benefits so that the buying power of the benefits does not diminish with inflation; and*
- *Take into account any potential effect on the Supplemental Security Income program when assessing the impact of any reform proposal. For example, if there are reductions in benefits for retirees and people with disabilities, under current law, the SSI program would have to step in to support many of those who would be forced further into poverty.*

H. Employment

1. Job training and vocational rehabilitation

On August 7, 1998, the President signed the Workforce Investment Act (WIA), which included the Rehabilitation Act Amendments of 1998. In the WIA, the employment and training provisions and adult literacy provisions specifically require that people with disabilities be considered a priority population for service delivery. *NCD commends Congress and the President for requiring the mainstream employment, training and literacy systems to prioritize service delivery to people with disabilities. This will enhance the likelihood that people with disabilities leaving the Temporary Assistance for Needy Families (TANF) rolls and the SSI/SSDI rolls will be able to access the services they need to obtain and retain competitive employment.*

NCD also commends congressional leaders who made the process of reauthorizing the act bipartisan and inclusive of the disability community. NCD praises Congress and the Administration for establishing better links between the vocational rehabilitation (VR) system and the general work force development system through this law. Jobseekers with disabilities will have improved options for service through the mainstream worker training and placement system, as well as through the disability-specific VR system. The U.S. Department of Labor has been providing valuable technical assistance to the network of one-stop career centers on how to provide nondiscriminatory and accessible services to people with disabilities. *While these preliminary efforts are a good start, the mainstream employment and training networks should implement a comprehensive training module so that line staff are well informed about resources available for people with disabilities seeking employment and are well equipped to meet the needs of clients with a wide range of disabilities.*

Perhaps the best improvement to the Rehabilitation Act in the WIA is the considerable strengthening of section 508, discussed in detail later in the technology section of this report. The U.S. Access Board has begun to develop the accessibility regulations, which are expected to have a major impact on the market availability of accessible technology, as industry designs products to meet federal procurement requirements.

Some other improvements to the Rehabilitation Act are worth noting. The Individual Plan for Employment (IPE) is the new term for the Individualized Written Rehabilitation Program (IWRP), which gives more control to consumers in developing their VR plan for services. VR plans may now be developed by the individual or an outside advocate, as long as the document is signed by a qualified rehabilitation counselor. The language is strengthened concerning the obligation of state VR agencies to offer informed choice to clients about service alternatives available to them, including those provided by other organizations both inside and outside the state. Trial work experiences are encouraged as a way for agencies to evaluate whether potential clients will benefit from VR assistance. States with an order of selection policy — by which persons with more severe disabilities receive priority for assistance — are nonetheless expected to provide core information and referral services to all people with disabilities who contact the agency within the state. Mediation is encouraged as an approach to resolving client-agency disputes without compromising the right to formal adjudication. The Rehabilitation Council, formerly Rehabilitation Advisory Council, has more of a role in developing agency policies and plans.

The Rehabilitation Act Amendments of 1998 were nonetheless disappointing in not going further in some areas. *The illogical division between the administration of VR services to people with visual disabilities and all other disabilities was not addressed. Stronger and more considered efforts should have been required to meet the needs of traditionally underserved populations, including people from diverse cultural communities, individuals with psychiatric disabilities, and residents of rural areas such as Indian reservations. State rehabilitation councils should have been given sign-off authority analogous to that which statewide independent living councils have on independent living plans. Client Assistance Programs should have been required to be independent from state VR agencies so they can advocate effectively from outside the VR system.*

In summary, the 1998 reauthorization of the Rehabilitation Act made some significant improvements but passed up an opportunity to make some important additional reforms. *NCD encourages the Rehabilitative Services Administration to work closely with the Presidential Task Force on Employment of Adults with Disabilities to develop bold, multiagency demonstration and research initiatives to achieve dramatically better outcomes in employment rates for people with disabilities, and to provide the policy options for a truly revolutionary reauthorization of the Rehabilitation Act that encompasses responses to the range of disincentives that have prevented people with disabilities seeking employment from succeeding. Moreover, NCD encourages the President and Congress to recognize that the VR program has received level funding for years and will require additional funding to adequately address the needs of people moving from welfare to work and from Social Security disability programs to work.*

2. Presidential task force on employment of adults with disabilities

As mentioned in the Introduction, President Clinton signed an executive order in March 1998 creating a task force chaired by the secretary of labor to develop policy recommendations for the President to bring the employment rate of adults with disabilities as close as possible to the level of the rest of the population. During the period covered in this report, the task force met twice and created a series of work groups to address specific employment topics listed in Section 2 of the executive order. A report including the outcome of the work group efforts and recommendations to the President was under development as the period covered by this progress report came to a close.

NCD commends the President for seeing the need to pull together a broad array of federal cabinet secretaries and agency heads to address what is clearly a multidimensional and challenging issue. As the work of the task force moves forward, NCD encourages the task force to recognize that some of the biggest barriers to employment for people with disabilities include work disincentives in our public benefit systems; the lack of accessible, affordable home- and community-based long-term services and supports; inadequate housing and transportation infrastructures; and a lack of educational credentials and work experience in the target population. Moreover, as long as students with disabilities drop out of high school at a rate twice that of their nondisabled peers, we will continue to see disappointing employment outcomes for young people with disabilities. Likewise, the unique needs of racial and ethnic minorities with disabilities in both the education and job training and rehabilitation systems must receive special attention so that the task force will reach the full population of adults with disabilities.

In short, NCD encourages the task force to take the opportunity the President has provided to develop broad-based, cross-cutting initiatives that will fundamentally alter the landscape of public policy for Americans with disabilities. The problem the task force has been asked to address will be solved only with dramatic, visionary approaches. Incremental tinkering with existing programs simply will not have the impact the President and the disability community want and need.

I. Welfare to work

1. Federal/state efforts

In the last year, a growing number of states, with support from federal partners, have recognized the need to address disability issues in their local welfare populations to achieve the desired outcomes of welfare reform. For example,

- Washington State finalized and released a validated screening tool for identifying people with learning disabilities in the welfare population.
- Arkansas became the first state to implement the use of the Washington State screen statewide.
- Kansas has implemented a statewide program to integrate adult literacy and welfare reform efforts for people with disabilities.
- Six of the welfare to work discretionary grants awarded by the Department of Labor (approximately $20 million in funding) went to local applicants who will use the money to address the needs of people with disabilities in their local welfare populations.
- In 1998, the National Institute for Literacy and the Office of Vocational and Adult Education at DOE funded four regional training and resource centers on learning disability issues for adults and required these centers to prioritize welfare reform issues for their target populations.

2. Increased federal funding

As part of the final budget approved at the end of the 105th Congress, a number of measures designed to expand welfare-to-work activities received funding. For example, the final budget included $283 million for 50,000 new vouchers exclusively for people who need housing assistance to make the transition from welfare to work. In addition, the budget included $75 million to assist states and localities in developing flexible transportation alternatives, such as van services, to help former welfare recipients and other low-income workers to get to work. It also included an extended welfare-to-work tax credit for employers as an incentive for them to hire, invest in training, and retain long-term welfare recipients. Similarly, the budget extended the work opportunity tax credit, which encourages employers to hire disadvantaged youth, welfare recipients, and qualified veterans. *NCD commends the President and Congress for recognizing the need to address housing, transportation, and other barriers to enable people on welfare to obtain and retain employment. NCD encourages the President and administering agencies for these new programs to recognize that a large percentage of the population remaining on TANF has disabilities ranging from learning disabilities to psychiatric disabilities to substance abuse issues. Accordingly, many of these individuals must have their disability-related needs addressed in order for the goal of obtaining long-term employment to be realized. Moreover, NCD encourages the President and Congress to recognize that the current efforts to move people from welfare to work may have important lessons for the growing effort to move people from reliance on disability benefit programs to employment. Issues like housing, transportation, and health care must be addressed for the SSI and SSDI populations as well if the transition to work is to be successful.*

J. Housing

For people with disabilities to achieve optimal employment outcomes, they must be able to find accessible, affordable housing with links to accessible, affordable transportation that will take them to their job. A number of significant actions took place in the last year that advanced housing policy for people with disabilities.

1. Definition of Housing for people with disabilities

HUD informed large cities and states that receive Community Development Block Grant (CDBG) and Housing Opportunities Made Equal (HOME) funds that people living in nursing homes and other service-centered facilities should be counted as being in need of permanent housing as opposed to being "housed." This statement is important because it recognizes the fact that institutional living does not constitute real housing for people with disabilities. It also will result in HUD receiving a more accurate and realistic count of the number of people with disabilities truly in need of housing. It is worth noting that even without this change in assessing the housing needs of people living in institutions, people with disabilities have been determined by HUD to be a population with the most urgent housing needs.

NCD commends HUD for taking steps to track more accurately the housing needs of people with disabilities. At the same time, NCD encourages HUD to act on its existing data and realign housing resources to respond more adequately to the appalling shortage in affordable, accessible housing in the community for people with disabilities. Moreover, NCD recommends that HUD further clarify its position on what constitutes housing for people with disabilities by issuing a policy statement to all recipients of HUD funds and placing the statement in fair housing materials and on its Web page.

2. Home purchase and renovations

On April 28, 1998, Fannie Mae announced the publication of *A Home of Your Own Guide*, the first manual specifically created to provide step-by-step homebuying guidance for people with disabilities. In early 1998, HUD included a disability rights organization (the Disability Rights Action Coalition for Housing) in a working group of major stakeholders in home ownership policy to implement a workable and effective home ownership program that will meet the needs of all people in the United States. Also, in early 1998, Secretary Andrew Cuomo issued a directive encouraging communities to use CDBG funds for home modifications for people with disabilities. *NCD commends Fannie Mae and HUD for taking these steps toward promoting homeownership and home modifications for people with disabilities. NCD encourages HUD to build on these steps by creating a national home modification fund for low- income people with disabilities, both renters and owners. HUD thereby will empower more people with disabilities to become homeowners or tenants in community settings.*

3. Visitability

In HUD's recent Notices of Funding Availability, the agency included bonus points for developers when they seek to build or rehabilitate structures with three or less units that include visitability by people with disabilities. This visitability concept would require all such new housing to have at least one no-step entrance and 32-inch doorways so people with disabilities could visit their friends who live there. In addition, at the same time, Secretary Cuomo issued a notice to all jurisdictions encouraging them to adopt visitability standards for all new construction projects, including town houses and single-family homes.

Last spring, the HOPE VI program (a HUD-financed effort to replace housing resources destroyed when public housing projects are demolished) issued a Notice of Funding Availability strongly encouraging applicants to incorporate both visitability and section 504 standards in new projects that would not be covered by the Fair Housing Act. All applications submitted in accordance with this NOFA included visitability and section 504 accessibility standards. *NCD commends HUD for embracing visitability as a goal for HUD-financed housing and for recognizing that the move from project-based housing to town homes and other detached dwellings does not need to mean a reduction in accessibility if developers are encouraged to build in such features in the design stage.*

4. Tenant-based rental assistance

Congress included $40 million in section 8 funding for people with disabilities, in part to offset the displacement likely to occur as a result of elderly-only designation of public housing formerly occupied by people with disabilities. *NCD applauds Congress for recognizing the need for substitute funding to enable low-income people with disabilities to find housing in the community, but believes HUD and Congress must go much further to expand funding for tenant-based rental certificates. In the past, HUD has used 25 percent of its section 811 program funds (Supportive Housing for People with Disabilities) for tenant-based rental certificates. NCD recommends that 100 percent of the section 811 program funds be used for person-based, rather than project-based, housing resources. This change would be consistent with the requirements in section 504 of the Rehabilitation Act and the Fair Housing Act that housing resources be provided in the most integrated setting appropriate.*

5. Task force on segregation and services linked to housing

One of the core debates within housing policy for people with disabilities centers on whether there are some circumstances under which people with disabilities may be required to live exclusively with other people with disabilities and/or to accept services in order to qualify for publicly funded housing. The resolution of this debate has important civil rights implications for people with disabilities, many of whom wish to live in integrated settings and to be able to seek services separate from their choice of where to live. For example, the Fair Housing Act and section 504 prohibit special terms and conditions and/or segregation based on disability status. Internally, HUD this fall created a Task Force on Segregation and Services Linked to Housing, which will examine ways to maximize integration and individual choice in housing for people with disabilities. *NCD is concerned that the issues of segregation and services linked to housing are well-decided under section 504 of the Rehabilitation Act and the Fair Housing Act. Accordingly, NCD does not understand the purpose of this new task force, unless it will focus exclusively on implementing well-established civil rights policies.*

6. Compliance with section 504 of the Rehabilitation Act by HUD and its grantees

Under section 504 of the Rehabilitation Act, public housing authorities must ensure that 5 percent of any building with five or more units is accessible to people with mobility impairments, and 2 percent of any such building is accessible for people with visual or hearing impairments. Recently, as more and more public housing authorities have reoriented their emphasis away from housing projects and toward low-density housing such as inaccessible town houses, the number of units accessible for people with disabilities has been significantly reduced.

NCD recommends that HUD conduct an evaluation of its grant recipients and subrecipients under section 504 of the Rehabilitation Act to ensure that all of their programs and services are in compliance. In conducting this evaluation, HUD is encouraged to move beyond a percentage mentality and promote the development and rehabilitation of housing that will meet the needs of all people.

Finally, NCD recommends that HUD reform the programs under which people with disabilities receive assistance with housing such as the section 811 program to ensure that these programs reflect the most integrated setting requirement of section 504 and independent living philosophy of the disability rights movement.

K. Transportation

Like housing, accessible and affordable transportation plays a vital role in enabling individuals with disabilities and their families to participate in the mainstream economic, social, and cultural lives of their communities.

1. Over-the-road bus regulations

This past year witnessed a significant step forward in transportation policy when DOT issued the final regulation implementing ADA provisions for over-the-road bus (OTRB) accessibility in September 1998. The regulation, widely regarded as a strong rule by the disability community, requires large fixed-route operators to achieve 50 percent of full fleet accessibility by October 2006 and 100 percent by October 2012. An important strength of the regulation is that it provides a regulatory definition of discriminatory action: refusing transportation, using or requesting the use of non-employees in giving routine assistance without the passenger's consent, and asking passengers to reschedule their trips to a time other than their requested travel time. Properly implemented, the regulation will make OTRB transportation accessible for people with mobility impairments for the first time since ADA was enacted. As written, however, the regulation both supports and detracts from ADA's overall goal for "fully accessible, nondiscriminatory, everyday service."

Small fixed-route carriers and those providing demand-responsive or mixed service have no minimum percentage of fleet accessibility to achieve. Instead, these carriers will be required only to provide an accessible bus on 48 hours' advance notice starting October 2001 (large carriers) or October 2002 (small carriers). New buses acquired by large fixed-route carriers after October 2000 must be accessible, while small carriers have no parallel requirement. Of 3,500 OTRB service providers, all but 21 are classified as small carriers. However, the major carriers serve the largest number of passengers.

Exempting most carriers from any minimum fleet accessibility requirement virtually guarantees that service to persons with disabilities will never be available on the same basis as to nondisabled passengers in many areas of the country. This outcome is not in keeping with the purposes of ADA. *Rather than accept less than full accessibility as the goal, NCD encourages DOT to find alternative paths for small operators to achieve full fleet accessibility over a longer time frame.*

DOT has strengthened the regulation by including provisions making OTRB operators individually and collectively accountable for providing accessible service. Each operator involved in providing service to passengers with disabilities on trips involving multiple transfers is responsible for communicating to ensure accessible service on all trip segments. Failures to provide the requested accessible service must be compensated at a rate ranging from $300 to $700. *NCD commends DOT for including provisions that clearly demonstrate its commitment to successful implementation of the regulation.*

NCD notes that a provision for DOT to conduct a regulatory review of all service requirements starting in October 2006 has positive and negative implications. On the positive side, DOT has set out the requirements it intends to reevaluate and what data it proposes to use. On the negative side is the possibility that the measurement data will not be maintained regularly and accurately. Without reliable data, DOT cannot make a fair assessment of the regulation's impact on the industry or the extent to which it has made OTRB transportation truly more accessible for people with disabilities. *NCD urges DOT to explore options and implement systems for ensuring the reliability of the data on which its analyses will depend.*

2. Air Carrier Access Act

The Air Carrier Access Act (ACAA), which became law in 1986, prohibits discrimination against passengers with disabilities by air carriers in providing air transportation services. The implementing regulation was passed in 1990. This year NCD conducted a study on DOT's enforcement of ACAA. The findings showed that DOT's enforcement model relies heavily on monitoring of complaints and voluntary compliance by air carriers. This approach does not emphasize traditional investigation and prosecution of complaints similar to other federal civil rights enforcement agencies.

Accordingly, NCD believes that DOT's approach is critically lacking in the key areas of compliance monitoring, complaint handling, and leadership. No regular program of ACAA monitoring ensures compliance in day-to-day airline operations. DOT's informal complaint- handling process serves more as a tool for monitoring the industry than as a system for resolving individual discrimination claims. Even the formal complaint process focuses only on issues of broad public interest, so that individual complainants have no reliable administrative means to obtain satisfaction unless the airline voluntarily cooperates. NCD's research shows that DOT's leadership in addressing difficult compliance problems (e.g., providing lifts and other boarding devices, regular training of airline personnel, and ensuring that new aircraft meet accessibility standards) has been inadequate.

The problems of ACAA enforcement arise from inadequacies in DOT's enforcement mechanism and in the law itself. Unlike other civil rights laws, ACAA does not explicitly establish a private right of action and contains no provisions for attorneys' fees and damages. The law also fails to extend the nondiscrimination mandate to foreign air carriers operating in the United States as code-sharing partners of domestic airlines. *NCD urges DOT to seek additional resources for enforcement of ACAA and to target specific areas where it will initiate action in concert with the disability community, the aviation industry, and other stakeholder groups to correct persistent implementation and compliance problems. NCD also encourages Congress to increase DOT's ACAA enforcement budget and to amend ACAA extending its nondiscrimination mandate to all airlines serving U.S. markets, strengthening DOT's enforcement mandate, and authorizing those whose civil rights have been violated to obtain appropriate legal remedies.*

L. Technology

Over the past year, several significant events have advanced the potential for individuals with disabilities to use the Internet and have access to the equipment they need to work, gain an education, and live independently. Of greatest significance are the changes to section 508 in the Rehabilitation Act Amendments of 1998, which strengthened the obligations of federal agencies to provide accessible technology and information to their employees, customers, and stakeholders.

1. Section 508 of the Rehabilitation Act

When section 508 was originally enacted in 1986, it required federal agencies to purchase office equipment that was accessible to its employees. However, no mechanism enforced this requirement. Furthermore, only technology manufacturers, and not individuals themselves, could file complaints. Now section 508 has been modified to grant authority to the Access Board for issuing accessibility regulations, which must be completed by February 7, 2000 (18 months after the amendments became law), and federal agencies must comply six months after that. Additionally, federal employees, as well as members of the public receiving services from the agency, now have the right to file a complaint under a procedure similar to that outlined under section 504 of the Rehabilitation Act.

Strong compliance with these regulations will have significant implications for people with disabilities who work for or receive services from the Federal Government and for the disability community at large. The Federal Government can use its considerable purchasing power to influence private industry toward developing universally designed technology that is accessible to everyone. One example of the impact of the Federal Government on technology development was the refusal of DOE to purchase Lotus Notes software until access modifications were made. Pursuant to DOE's software procurement policy, which was developed in consultation with experts in accessible software standards, DOE will not purchase any software product for use by its employees that does not meet minimal accessibility standards. For example, to meet such standards, software must be completely operable with keyboard commands rather than requiring mouse navigation; must allow for compatibility with screen reader and voice input programs; and must have accessible product support, including accessible documentation, training materials, and technical support. DOE's insistence on access has led to the development of more accessible Lotus products. *NCD encourages other agencies to take their example from DOE and adopt its accessible software procurement standards during the period while the section 508 accessibility standards are being developed.*

2. Section 255 of the Telecommunications Act

Another significant technology development this year was the issuance of proposed regulations to implement Section 255 of the Telecommunications Act of 1996. This law requires that telecommunications equipment and services be accessible to individuals with disabilities, where readily achievable. In June, the Federal Communications Commission (FCC) proposed rules to implement this section of the Act. *While NCD was pleased that FCC proposed these overdue regulations, and that Chairman William Kennard has publicly expressed support for the development of accessible technology, NCD is disappointed that FCC is considering such a narrow definition of "telecommunications." It is astounding that voice mail, faxes, e-mail, and other commonly used electronic communications tools may not be covered. Such a narrow definition seems at odds with the intent of Congress and a common sense understanding of telecommunications in the 1990s and beyond. The failure to regulate even the most commonly used forms of telecommunications will result in the exclusion of people with sensory and other impairments from basic communications devices and services, to say nothing of those yet to emerge from the rapidly changing Information Age.*

3. ADA and section 504 of the Rehabilitation Act

Prior to the period covered in this report, Congress enacted other laws to ensure information access to individuals with disabilities, including Titles II and III of ADA and section 504 of the Rehabilitation Act. Unfortunately, federal agencies with enforcement authority for these laws have lagged behind in their compliance monitoring. In particular, the DOJ has failed to issue any advisory guidance on access to information kiosks operated by units of state and local government and has not issued significant guidance or consent decrees related to technology access. Only in September 1998 did DOJ assign a specific individual from its Disability Rights Section the responsibility to develop expertise in technology issues. *NCD urges DOJ to prioritize technology-access issues in its implementation of ADA.*

4. Assistive Technology Act

For the past ten years, DOE has funded projects at the state level to promote systems change and advocacy activities that enhance access of children and adults with disabilities to assistive technology devices and services. These projects were authorized under the Technology-Related Assistance for Individuals with Disabilities Act. In October 1998, Congress passed a law called the Assistive Technology Act. This law continues block grants to states for public education and advocacy related to assistive technology products and services. In addition, the law authorizes a new micro loan program to encourage the development and purchase of accessible technology-related products and services. *NCD is disappointed that more emphasis was not given to promoting universal design or built-in accessibility, as contrasted with assistive technology or add-on accessibility. The rapid rate of technological change makes it increasingly difficult for compatible assistive technology to be developed before new versions of related mainstream products are released on the market. In addition, NCD recommends that more be done to promote training on use of the Internet, such as through public libraries, because of its revolutionary potential to empower people with various disabilities in education, employment, and civic activities. Independent, consumer-driven evaluations of technology also should have been specifically encouraged, since consumers face a bewildering array of options and have difficulty making informed decisions based mainly on product marketing literature. Finally, since people with disabilities and their families are disproportionately poor, it is critical that technology resources be affordable or available in free, accessible public venues if the disability community is to keep pace with the Information Age.*

M. International issues

As ADA continues to serve as a model of civil rights legislation for countries throughout the world, there is strong international interest in how ADA implementation is proceeding. NCD remains confident that the results of our ADA monitoring project will continue to attract interest. In the interim, the last year witnessed significant developments in the international arena.

1. Organization of American States

The Organization of American States (OAS) continues to consider the "Inter-American Convention on the Elimination of All Forms of Discrimination by Reason of Disability." This convention, when passed, will create an opportunity for OAS to carry out a great responsibility to ensure that all its state members observe the convention. *NCD encourages the U.S. Permanent Mission to the Organization of American States to work to see that the Convention is adopted with strong antidiscrimination provisions and to advocate that the Convention be fully implemented by each State Member when it is passed. In addition, NCD again commends the Department of State, including the U.S. Organization of American States, for its efforts to involve NCD and other disability community stakeholders in reviewing draft policies.*

2. Department of State

NCD encourages the Department of State to take steps to ensure that all aspects of U.S. foreign policy and assistance recognize the human rights and civil rights of all people with disabilities, by ensuring compliance with the Architectural Barriers Act, Section 504 of the Rehabilitation Act, and ADA in U.S. embassies, consular offices, missions, and other U.S.-owned or leased property abroad; including relevant information about the status of people with disabilities abroad in U.S. government-generated country reports; promoting democracy through the sharing of U.S. laws and policies that promote inclusion, independence and empowerment; and conducting self-evaluations under the Rehabilitation Act for all U.S. government agencies active abroad to identify barriers to participation by qualified people with disabilities and to establish transition plans to eliminate these barriers.

Similarly, NCD encourages the Department of State and the United States Agency for International Development to ensure that all foreign aid and assistance is developed and delivered in a manner that ensures full participation and accessi-bility by all people with disabilities and their families in the geographic region served by the aid or assistance. If this practice were followed, the United States would not have recently permitted Bosnia to use U.S. aid to purchase thousands of dollars worth of inaccessible buses. Finally, NCD encourages the Department of State to take steps to ensure that people with disabilities are a significant part of the work force at all levels of domestic and international operations by U.S. agencies handling international activities.

Conclusion

Increasing the employment rate of people with disabilities and expanding choices in home- and community-based long-term services and supports are two of the most significant issues in disability policy today. Neither of these issues is subject to quick and cheap solutions. Both require bold steps by the President and Congress, and both require multifaceted solutions. On the employment front, it is critical to recognize that early intervention and life-long development of human capital must be part of the solution. For children with disabilities, employment goals should be established early in their educations, and the development of marketable skills must be emphasized in the classroom and in work-study placements. People who acquire disabil-ities as adults must receive the comprehensive medical and vocation reha-bilitation they need in a timely manner, coupled with access to accessible and affordable transportation and housing and a technological infrastructure that will ease the transition back to employment.

On the issue of long-term services and supports, including consumer-directed personal assistance services and family supports such as respite care, the President and Congress must recognize that children and adults with significant disabilities and their families can contribute more to the economy and enjoy a basic standard of living taken for granted by many in the rest of the population if we eliminate the institutional bias in Med-icaid and require states to honor the human rights of their citizens with disabilities to live where they choose, with adequate supports to participate fully in community life. Finally, for both the employment issue and the long-term services and supports issue to be addressed effectively, the Pres-ident and Congress must work together to remove the work disincentives from our Social Security, Medicaid, and Medicare systems. Americans with disabilities are poised to take their place in the mainstream of their com-munities, but they are too often thwarted in this desire by outdated federal policies and programs. Now is the time for the President and Congress to carry out President Bush's promise that people with disabilities be given "the opportunity to blend fully and equally into the right mosaic of the American mainstream."

References

1. The Web site address is http://www.infouse.com/disabilitydata. The information contained there is excerpted from Stoddard, S., Jans, L., Ripple, J., and Kraus, L. (1998). *Chartbook on Work and Disability in the United States, 1998.* An InfoUse Report. Washington, D.C.: U.S. National Institute on Disability and Rehabilitation Research.

2. Data reported last year by the U.S. Bureau of the Census based on *Survey of Income and Program Participation* results from 1994 indicated that 54 million people of all ages reported having a disability, 26 million of whom said that their disability was severe.

3. Some researchers have pointed out that the relatively low rates of disability in the Asian Pacific Islander and Hispanic communities may stem from a reluctance of recent immigrants with disabilities in these groups to self-identify on surveys, either because of unusually negative cultural associations with disability or because of fear of their disability status being used to undermine their ability to remain in the United States. See, for example, Leung, Paul. 1992. Asian Pacific Americans and Section 21 of the Rehabilitation Act Amendments of 1992. *American Rehabilitation,* 22(1): 2-6.

4. Note that measurements of activity limitation in children do not capture the full range of impairment and disability in children. For example, many children served under the Individuals with Disabilities Education Act, particularly children with mental disabilities, may not show up on surveys that narrowly ask about activity limitations.

5. For a more thorough discussion of this topic, see NCD's 1998 publication, *Reorienting Disability Research,* at http://www.ncd.gov.

6. For a thorough discussion of assisted suicide from a disability perspective, see NCD's 1997 publication, *Assisted Suicide: A Disability Perspective,* available on our Web site at http://www.ncd.gov.

7. The report, entitled *Grassroots Experiences with Government Programs and Disability Policy,* is available from NCD's Web site at http://www.ncd.gov.

8. *National Council on Disability, Removing Barriers to Work: Action Proposals for the 105th Congress and Beyond,* September 24, 1997.

Appendix C

Assisted suicide: a disability perspective

Professor Robert L. Burgdorf, Jr.
University of the District of Columbia School of Law

Written for the National Council on Disability.
Reproduced with Permission of the National Council on Disability.
Marca Bristo, Chairperson
Last Updated: September 14, 1998

Executive summary

Physician-assisted suicide and related issues have garnered much judicial, media, and scholarly attention in recent months. Two cases presently pending before the United States Supreme Court raise the issue of the legality of state laws prohibiting physician-assisted suicide. As the principal agency within the federal government charged with the responsibility of providing cross-disability policy analysis and recommendations regarding government programs and policies that affect people with disabilities, the National Council on Disability is issuing this position paper in the hope of presenting a coherent and principled stance on these issues drawn from the input and viewpoints of individuals with disabilities.

In the body of this position paper, the Council examines a number of insights derived from the experiences of people with disabilities focusing on the following topics:

- The Paramount Issue — Rights, Services, and Options
- The Reality and Prevalence of Discrimination
- Deprivation of Choices and the Importance of Self-Determination

- Others' Underestimation of Life Quality
- Fallibility of Medical Predictions
- Eschewing the Medical Model of Disabilities
- The Impact of Onset of Disability Upon Emotional State and Decision-Making
- The Reality of Living with Pain and Bodily Malfunction
- Divergent Interests of Those Involved in Assisted Suicide Decisions

Based upon these insights from those who have experienced disabilities and upon the existing legal framework, the National Council on Disability has formulated its position on the issue of physician-assisted suicide for persons with imminently terminal conditions as follows:

> *The benefits of permitting physician-assisted suicide are substantial and should not be discounted; they include respect for individual autonomy, liberty, and the right to make one's own choices about matters concerning one's intimate personal welfare; affording the dignity of control and choice for a patient who otherwise has little control of her or his situation; allowing the patient to select the time and circumstances of death rather than being totally at the mercy of the terminal medical condition; safeguarding the doctor/patient relationship in making this final medical decision; giving the patient the option of dying in an alert condition rather than in a medicated haze during the last hours of life; and, most importantly, giving the patient the ability to avoid severe pain and suffering.*

The Council finds, however, that at the present time such considerations are outweighed by other weighty countervailing realities. The benefits of physician-assisted suicide only apply to the small number of people who actually have an imminently terminal condition, are in severe, untreatable pain, wish to commit suicide, and are unable to do so without a doctor's involvement.

The dangers of permitting physician-assisted suicide are immense. The pressures upon people with disabilities to choose to end their lives, and the insidious appropriation by others of the right to make that choice for them are already prevalent and will continue to increase as managed health care and limitations upon health care resources precipitate increased "rationing" of health care services and health care financing.

People with disabilities are among society's most likely candidates for ending their lives, as society has frequently made it clear that it believes they would be better off dead, or better that they had not been born. The experience in the Netherlands demonstrates that legalizing assisted suicide generates strong pressures upon individuals and families to utilize that option, and leads very quickly to coercion and involuntary euthanasia. If assisted suicide were to become legal, the lives of people with any disability deemed too difficult to live with would be at risk, and persons with disabilities who are poor or members of racial minorities would likely be in the most jeopardy of all.

If assisted suicide were to be legalized, the only way to ward off the most dire ramifications for people with disabilities would be to create stringent procedural prerequisites. But, to be effective, such procedural safeguards would necessarily sacrifice individual autonomy to the supervision of medical and legal overlords to an unacceptable degree — the cure being as bad as the disease.

For many people with disabilities, it is more often the discrimination, prejudice, and barriers that they encounter, and the restrictions and lack of options that this society has imposed, rather than their disabilities or their physical pain, that cause people-with-disabilities' lives to be unsatisfactory and painful. The notion that a decision to choose assisted suicide must be preceded by a full explanation of the programs, resources, and options available to assist the patient if he or she does not decide to pursue suicide, strikes *many* people with disabilities as a very shallow promise when they know that all too often the programs are too few, the resources are too limited, and the options are nonexistent. Society should not be ready to give up on the lives of its citizens with disabilities until it has made real and persistent efforts to give these citizens a fair and equal chance to achieve a meaningful life.

For these reasons, the Council has decided that at this time in the history of American society it opposes the legalization of assisted suicide. Current evidence indicates clearly that the interests of the few people who would benefit from legalizing physician-assisted suicide are heavily outweighed by the probability that any law, procedures, and standards that can be imposed to regulate physician-assisted suicide will be misapplied to unnecessarily end the lives of people with disabilities, and entail an intolerable degree of intervention by legal and medical officials in such decisions. On balance, the current illegality of physician-assisted suicide is preferable to the limited benefits to be gained by its legalization. At least until such time as our society provides a comprehensive, fully funded, and operational system of assistive-living services for people with disabilities, this is the only position that the National Council on Disability can, in good conscience, support.

I. Introduction

Physician-assisted suicide and related issues have garnered much judicial, media, and scholarly attention in recent months. Well-publicized instances of legal prosecutions of medical practitioners, such as Dr. Jack Kevorkian, for engaging in acts of assisted suicide, and recent consideration by the United States Supreme Court of a pair of cases in which the legality of state laws prohibiting physicians from assisting suicides by their patients has been contested, have generated considerable debate, controversy, and pontificating by various individuals and organizations.

As the principal agency within the federal government charged with the responsibility of providing cross-disability policy analysis and recommendations regarding government programs and policies that affect people with disabilities, the National Council on Disability is issuing this position paper in the hope of presenting a coherent and principled stance on these issues, drawn from the input and sometimes conflicting viewpoints of individuals with disabilities. This position paper was drafted for the National Council on Disability by Professor Robert L. Burgdorf, Jr., of the University of the District of Columbia School of Law.

II. Complexity of the issues

Discussions of the issues surrounding the question of physician-assisted suicide should not oversimplify the subject. While various individuals and organizations have sometimes formulated their positions in ways that make the issues seem simple and straightforward, consideration of the legal, medical, and societal implications of assisted suicide are inherently thorny and multifaceted. If one limits consideration only to matters of legality, the question, whether or not physician-assisted suicide should be legal, involves a number of component questions: Is there or should there be a legal right to commit suicide? Should it ever be legal for some other person to assist in a suicide? Should a physician ever be permitted to assist in a suicide? Should any right to commit suicide or to assist in someone else's suicide be limited to situations where a person is terminally ill? If so, how imminent must the person's death be? Should any right to commit suicide or to assist in someone else's suicide be limited to situations where a person is in severe pain? If so, how much pain suffices? Sporadic or constant pain? What if the pain is partially or fully treatable? Is it assisting suicide to treat pain with medication or other techniques that will shorten life? Should a person's age and life expectancy ever be considered? Is there a difference in the criteria that should be applied to determinations whether or not to provide ordinary medical treatment; to provide, refuse to provide, or to terminate "extraordinary measures"; or to assist the termination or shortening of life? Should there be a difference in the requirements and standards applied to decisions to administer medical procedures that will save a person's life versus those that will merely extend it somewhat? Who should make such determinations—the patient, the doctor, the family, medical review boards, the courts? Do the same or different considerations apply regarding individuals who are not capable of making the decisions about their treatment themselves? What types of procedural safeguards should be imposed to ensure the integrity of the decision-making process? Can such procedural prerequisites be workable and effective in application?

Even the more straightforward situation where an individual is able to take her or his own life without direct assistance involves its own legal complications. If a physician prescribes medication that is used in the suicide, the doctor may risk legal liability to the extent that it appears that the doctor intentionally prescribed the medication for that purpose. And the individual who decides to take his or her life may endanger family members or others who are present when the deed is done, because they may risk liability for aiding or abetting the suicide, a circumstance that at the very least adds stress, guilt, or isolation and loneliness for all of those involved in the scenario.

This position paper does not aim to unravel all such complexities and answer all of the foregoing questions. It seeks, rather, to delineate some criteria and principles derived from the experiences and deliberations of people with disabilities that will hopefully enlighten future initiatives undertaken by the federal government and the states to refine the law in this area. There can be little question that current laws and legal principles regarding treatment, non-treatment, and assisted suicide need refinement. One of the ironies of the law as it currently stands has been described by a physician in an article in the *New England Journal of Medicine* in which he cited two hypothetical patients:

> *One is 28 years old, despondent over the recent breakup of a romantic relationship, and because of an acute asthma attack, temporarily dependent on a ventilator. Apart from asthma, this person is in good health. The other patient is 82 years old, is wracked with pain from extensive metastic cancer, and has only a few weeks to live. Assume that both persons want to end their lives, the 28-year-old by refusing the ventilator and the 82-year-old by suicide. Under current law, the 28-year-old has the right to refuse the ventilator, whereas the 82-year-old generally lacks the right to assistance with suicide.[1]*

People with disabilities report numerous other problems with the law as it currently stands, including unconsented denials of treatment, pressure to refuse or discontinue treatments, disregard of requests for relief from pain, "Do-Not-Resuscitate" consent forms hidden within a stack of admission and consent papers, and involuntary assisted "suicide."

III. The cases under consideration by the Supreme Court

The United States Supreme Court has before it this term two cases that raise the question of the legality of physician suicide and the permissibility of state laws that prohibit it — *Vacco v. Quill*[2] and *State of Washington v. Glucksberg*.[3] This section provides a brief summary of those two cases. As a precedential backdrop, however, it is important to be aware of a prior decision of the Court — *Cruzan v. Director, Mo. Dept. of Health*.[4]

In *Cruzan*, the Court considered the challenge by the parents of a woman who had been in a coma for seven years following an automobile accident to the refusal by state hospital officials and the Missouri Supreme Court to authorize the removal of a feeding tube keeping Nancy Cruzan alive. The Supreme Court of the United States upheld Missouri's legal standard for such cases, which required "clear and convincing evidence" of the patient's wishes before life support could be removed. In doing so, the Court recognized that "a competent person has a constitutionally protected liberty interest in refusing unwanted medical treatment", and assumed for the purposes of the case that the Constitution "would grant a competent person a constitutionally protected right to refuse lifesaving hydration and nutrition."

In its reasoning upholding the Missouri legal framework restricting the removal of life support for persons not able to make the decision themselves, the *Cruzan* Court recognized Missouri's interests in the protection and preservation of life and in avoiding erroneous decisions to withdraw life-sustaining treatment. It noted in passing that "the majority of States in this country have laws imposing criminal penalties on one who assists another to commit suicide."

The current cases examine the legality of such state laws. The *Vacco* and *Glucksberg* cases present the Court with two different legal theories under which physician-assisted suicide laws have been challenged — in *Vacco*, equal protection, and in *Glucksberg*, due process.

In *Vacco v. Quill*,[5] three terminally ill patients and three physicians who treat terminally ill patients, challenged the constitutionality of New York statutes that made it a crime (manslaughter) for any person to intentionally cause or aid another to commit suicide. The plaintiffs challenged the laws as violating both the due-process and equal-protection guarantees of the U.S. Constitution. The trial court dismissed both claims. On appeal, the United States Court of Appeals for the Second Circuit ruled that the N.Y. assisted-suicide laws violated the Equal Protection Clause because they are not rationally related to any legitimate state interest.[6] In reaching this conclusion, the Second Circuit reasoned as follows:

> *New York does not treat similarly circumstanced persons alike: those in the final stages of terminal illness who are on life-support systems are allowed to hasten their deaths by directing the removal of such systems; but those who are similarly situated, except for the previous attachment of life-sustaining equipment, are not allowed to hasten death by self-administering prescribed drugs.*[7]

The Second Circuit found that there was no legitimate state interest to support the difference in treatment between terminally ill patients on life-support and those seeking assistance in directly ending their lives. The Supreme Court agreed to review the Second Circuit's equal protection ruling in *Vacco*.

State of Washington v. Glucksberg[8] involves a similar challenge, by four physicians who treat terminally ill patients, three terminally ill persons, and an organization that provides assistance to terminally ill persons, to the constitutionality of a Washington law that makes it a crime for any person

who knowingly causes or aids another person to attempt suicide. The plaintiffs had challenged the Washington statute under the Equal Protection and
Due Process clauses of the U.S. Constitution. The district court granted
summary judgment in favor of the plaintiffs on both claims.

A panel of the United States Court of Appeals for the Ninth Circuit
initially reversed the decision on both grounds, but on rehearing en banc,
the Ninth Circuit ruled that the Washington statute violates due process. It
began its analysis by finding that there is a constitutionally protected liberty
interest "in choosing the time and manner of one's death," and more particularly that "[a] competent terminally ill adult, having lived nearly the full
measure of his life, has a strong liberty interest in choosing a dignified and
humane death rather than being reduced at the end of his existence to a
childlike state of helplessness, diapered, sedated, incontinent."

The Ninth Circuit then weighed these liberty interests of the terminally
ill patient against the state's interests in preserving life, preventing suicide,
in avoiding the taking of life due to "a fit of desperation, depression, or
loneliness or as a result of any other problem, physical or psychological,
which can be significantly ameliorated," and in avoiding deaths resulting
from undue influence by family members and physicians. The Ninth Circuit
ruled that some of these interests were diminished because the patient's life
was going to end anyway, and that the others could be better served
"through procedural safeguards, rather than through a complete ban on
assisted suicide."

The Supreme Court agreed to review the Second Circuit's due process
ruling in *Glucksberg*. The Court heard oral arguments on the *Vacco* and
Glucksberg cases on January 8, 1997.

IV. Perspectives of individuals with disabilities

Many people are interested in the subject of assisted suicide. Many in the
medical profession, including physicians, nurses, and hospital administrators have spoken out about their views on these matters, and the American
Medical Association has taken a position. Ethicists and religious officials
have articulated their analyses. Organizations for and against assisted suicide have advocated for their respective positions. Family members of persons with terminal illnesses have had strong feelings on these issues. The
courts, including the Supreme Court of the United States, have increasingly
been asked to address these types of issues.

Another group whose constituents often have strong views about
assisted suicide is people with disabilities. Given that persons suffering from
terminal illnesses and those experiencing severe pain almost always meet
the definition of individuals with disabilities, and that people with disabilities run the risk of being subject to life-shortening measures even when they
may not in fact have life-threatening conditions, the views and insights of
people with disabilities would seem to be very significant to the debate on
this issue. And yet the viewpoints of individuals with disabilities have been,

if not ignored, at least not a major piece of the public and judicial debate on this issue.

In submitting *amicus curiae* briefs in the two Supreme Court cases addressing physician-assisted suicide cases, the solicitor general and Department of Justice attorneys were required to identify the interests of the United States in the litigation that justified its involvement in the cases. In its briefs, the United States pointed to two such interests — the fact that the United States owns and operates health care facilities (such as V.A. hospitals and nursing homes), and the fact that federal law requires health care providers receiving Medicaid and Medicare funds to inform patients that they have a right to refuse life-sustaining treatment and to record any directives in this regard they may have. Seemingly much more directly relevant, but not mentioned in the briefs, is the fact that under the federal Rehabilitation Act and the Americans with Disabilities Act the United States, through the Department of Justice, is responsible for enforcement of requirements that people with disabilities not be discriminated against by federal, state, and private hospitals and other health care providers. This duty of ensuring that people with disabilities are treated equally in regard to medical treatment is not relied upon, nor even mentioned, in the Department of Justice briefs.

A. A Split of Opinion?

Within the disability community, divergent opinions about assisted suicide have given rise to heated debates; advocates for the differing positions articulate strong arguments that theirs is the more informed position or is more representative of a majority of individuals with disabilities. The absence of a single consensus viewpoint within the group does not mean, however, that the opposing views cancel one another out; each of the viewpoints is significant. The two separate points of view in the disability community are each voicing a legitimate and weighty concern that is rooted in the disability experience.

On the one hand, those individuals with disabilities, and organizations who favor assisted suicide help to point out that people with disabilities are entitled to, and in the past have often been deprived of, the opportunity to make full choices for themselves. Individuals with disabilities should be entitled, says this view, to make their own life choices without interference from medical personnel and society at large, particularly when the choice is one to avoid unbearable pain by foregoing a few days, weeks, or months of additional life. Other members of the disability community and organizations representing them argue that assisted suicide has been and will be used to cut short the lives of people with disabilities whose quality of life and worth as human beings have long been egregiously undervalued by society. Each of these viewpoints has considerable basis in truth. And both of them are motivated by an underlying desire that people with disabilities be accorded a position of dignity and equality in American society. The National

Council on Disability believes that articulating with more particularity the various insights of people with disabilities that bear upon the decisions whether or not to prolong, and whether or not to abet, the shortening of life of individuals with serious medical conditions, will provide considerable guidance and enlightenment as to how these issues should be resolved and the way laws ought to address such matters in the future.

B. Insights from the disability experience

1. The paramount issue — rights, services, and options
   Arguments for or against assisted suicide in particular situations are often framed in terms of future quality of life of the affected individual. These appraisals of life quality of people with disabilities occur in a context — the opportunities, impediments, services, burdens, rights, responsibilities, pleasures, suffering, assistance, and obstacles that the individual can expect in her or his situation in our society. In large part, this context is defined by society's treatment of people with disabilities — the barriers it has erected or tolerated, or prohibited and removed; the rights it has recognized and enforced, or denied, ignored, or not implemented; the services it has provided or fostered, or refused or neglected to provide; the independence and options it has conferred and promoted, or the dependence it has accepted and perpetuated; the suffering it has allowed or condoned, or addressed and ameliorated; the isolation and invisibility it has imposed or accepted, or the integration and participation it has instilled; the choices it has enabled and respected, or its withdrawal of the very liberty to make choices or acquiescence to the absence of any real choices.

   The National Council believes that the issue of assisted suicide should be viewed as interrelated with more basic, general issues of the rights, opportunities, and status of people with disabilities in our nation, and of the services, programs, policies, options, and choices our society makes available for people with disabilities. In its July 1996 report to the President and the Congress, *Achieving Independence: The Challenge for the 21st Century,* the Council presented over 120 recommendations addressing 11 broad topic areas for improving laws, policies, programs, and services for people with disabilities. Implementing the recommendations in *Achieving Independence* would go a long way toward assuring that any self-assessment or decision about the quality of life of an individual with a disability would be made in an optimal context of independence, equality of opportunity, full participation, and empowerment.

   In addition, people with terminal illnesses would benefit greatly from expanded availability of hospice services. These programs provide a team-oriented program of care that seeks to treat and comfort persons with terminal conditions in their homes or in home-like settings, with an emphasis on pain management and control of symptoms.[9] They seek to ameliorate the psychological, spiritual, and physical pain that may be associated with the process of dying, and they provide support for family members and friends while their loved one is dying, and bereavement care after the person has died.[10] More than 90% of hospice care hours are provided in patients' homes, thus substituting for more expensive and more disorienting hospitalization.[11] Studies indicate great savings in hospice costs versus alternative forms of treatment.[12] And yet such programs are not yet as widely available as they need to be.[13]

People with disabilities have long tried to convince the rest of society that the most serious problems facing those who have disabilities often arise, not from the disability itself, but from societal attitudes toward and treatment of individuals with disabilities. In 1975, a United Nations Expert Group declared that:

> *Despite everything we can do, or hope to do, to assist each physically or mentally disabled person achieve his or her maximum potential in life, our efforts will not succeed until we have found the way to remove the obstacles to this goal directed by human society — the physical barriers we have created in public buildings, housing, transportation, houses of worship, centers of social life, and other community facilities — the social barriers we have evolved and accepted against those who vary more than a certain degree from what we have been conditioned to regard as normal. More people are forced into limited lives and made to suffer by these man-made obstacles than by any specific physical or mental disability.[14]*

This idea that external factors are more damaging than the characteristics of disability itself is an important insight in trying to evaluate options for dealing with the impact of medical conditions and living with impairments. It suggests that people are likely to have much more success in dealing with their disabilities if they are informed about accommodations and services they may be able to use, and if there are sufficient support services and resources in place to assist in the individual's efforts to cope with the situation. In one dramatic example, Larry McAfee, a Georgia man who was involved in a motorcycle accident that left him quadriplegic and dependent on a ventilator, went to court to establish his right to discontinue the ventilator with the expectation that he would die.[15] Publicity about the case led, however, to communications with disability advocates and an outpouring of community support. Buoyed by this information and support, McAfee refused to exercise his court-recognized "right to die," fought to be released from a nursing home, and got himself a job.

The *McAfee* outcome is in stark contrast with the situation of Kenneth Bergstedt who, with disabilities similar to McAfee's, had his ventilator discontinued and died, principally because he feared being forced to live in a nursing home after the death of his father. The Nevada Supreme Court, ruling after Bergstedt's death, concluded that his "suffering resulted more from his fear of the unknown than any source of physical pain," and noted that he did not have a realistic understanding of his options sufficient to make an intelligent life-or-death decision.[16] Reviewing the limited assistance afforded Bergstedt before his death, a dissenting judge commented: "With this kind of support it is no wonder that he decided to do himself in."[17] If he were still alive, said the court, "it would have been necessary to fully inform him of the care alternatives that would have been available to him after his father's death or incapacity."[18]

The *Bergstedt* situation focuses on patients being provided accurate information about services, support, and other resources. Equally, or more important, however, is that adequate support systems and options be in place and available. People with disabilities facing medical treatment decisions need both information about options and the availability of the options themselves. Such community support services may take a variety of forms — counseling, independent-living services, vocational rehabilitation, treatment of depression, contact with disability peers and organizations, clear and understandable medical information, financial resources, housing options, transportation options, assistive devices, interpreters and personal care assistance, various types of therapy, job training, and others.

Clearly the elimination of discriminatory barriers and the availability of support services and financial resources, including adequate health insurance, will greatly impact the chances that a person will successfully deal with a disability. In the final analysis, most people with disabilities would welcome the same amount of attention for community support services and resources, and the kinds of efforts recommended in *Achieving Independence* as is currently being focused on the issue of assisted suicide.

2. The Reality and prevalence of discrimination

The opposing views within the disability community on the issue of assisted suicide share a common ground — a recognition of the danger of discrimination to the interests and fair treatment of people with disabilities. Those opposed to assisted suicide fear that deeply ingrained prejudice and patterns of undervaluing the worth of individuals having disabilities have led and will predictably continue to lead to the unnecessary deaths of persons with disabilities. Those who believe that people with disabilities should have access to physician-assisted suicide point out that one of the principle dynamics that has prevented people with disabilities from occupying a position of equality and dignity in society has been the denial of the right of people with disabilities to make their own choices, and that other people have often imposed undesired life choices upon people with disabilities.

Neither point of view doubts the existence of discrimination against people with disabilities.

On many previous occasions, the Council has discussed and documented the existence of widespread and virulent discrimination on the basis of disability. The existence of such discrimination and the deleterious effect that it has upon citizens with disabilities and our nation were primary reasons that in 1986 the Council proposed the enactment of the Americans with Disabilities Act (ADA). In enacting the ADA, Congress expressly found that "historically, society has tended to isolate and segregate individuals with disabilities, and despite some improvements, such forms of discrimination continue to be a serious and pervasive social problem."[19] Further, it declared that individuals with disabilities "have been faced with restrictions and limitations, subjected to a history of purposeful unequal treatment, and relegated to a position of political powerlessness in our society.[20] Congress also made findings that such discrimination persists in the critical areas of "health services ... and access to public services."[21] Discrimination against people with disabilities in regard to medical treatment had previously examined by the U.S. Commission on Civil Rights which concluded that people with disabilities "face discrimination in the availability and delivery of medical services" including the "withholding of lifesaving medical treatment."[22] The deep-seated nature of discrimination on the basis of disability has been widely acknowledged and documented by numerous other authorities.[23] Discrimination against them because of their disabilities is a daily experience of many individuals with disabilities.

3. Deprivation of choices and the importance of self-determination

Many people with disabilities subscribe to an approach to living with disabilities that is termed "independent living." The Council has endorsed the independent-living philosophy and it has been embraced in various federal statutes.[24] The U.S. Commission on Civil Rights has observed that a key element of independent living is self-determination for individuals with disabilities: "Independent-living programs insist on 'client self-choice rather than incorporation of the client into a set of goals established by program managers, service professionals, or funding mechanisms....'"[25] At the core of the independent living philosophy is a conviction that people with disabilities "desire to lead the fullest lives possible, outside of institutions, integrated into the community, exercising full freedom of choice."[26] One disability advocate has elaborated:

> *"Independent living is ...to live where and how one chooses and can afford. It is living within the community in the neighborhood one chooses. It is living alone or with a roommate of one's choice. It is deciding one's own pattern of life-schedule, food, entertainment, vices, virtues, leisure, and friends. It is freedom to take risks and freedom to make mistakes."[27]*

Regarding the latter point, some authorities have described the "dignity of risk," a concept that counters overprotection of people with disabilities by advocating a right of such people to take normal risks.[28] One commentator has observed: "The dignity of risk is what the independent living movement is all about. Without the possibility of failure, the disabled person is said to lack true independence and the mark of ones humanity — the right to choose for good or evil."[29]

1992 amendments to the Rehabilitation Act increased the focus on independent living and spelled out in more detail the approach that Congress understood to be represented by that phrase. Congress found that:

> *Disability is a normal part of the human experience and in no way diminishes the right of individuals to — (A) live independently; (B) enjoy self-determination; (C) make choices; (D) contribute to society; (E) pursue meaningful careers; and (F) enjoy full inclusion and integration in the economic, political, social, cultural, and educational mainstream of American society.*[30]

Congress also declared that "the goals of the nation properly include the goal of providing individuals with disabilities with the tools necessary to — (A) make informed choices and decisions; and (B) achieve…independent living …for such individuals."[31] However phrased, it is clear that equality and dignity for people with disabilities are strongly connected to the ability to of individuals with disabilities to make important life choices for themselves.

4. Others' underestimation of life quality

One of the hallmarks of societal attitudes toward disabilities has been a tendency of people without disabilities to overestimate the negative aspects and underestimate the positive features of the lives of those who have disabilities. The attitude of "I don't see how you can live with that" — sometimes expressed more dramatically as "I'd rather be dead than have [X disability]" — is one that people often exhibit in their encounters with people with disabilities.

The U.S. Commission on Civil Rights has described the "extremely extensive" negative connotations of disability: "To the fact that a [person with a disability] differs from the norm physically or mentally, people often add a value judgment that such a difference is a big and very negative one."[32] The United States Supreme Court has acknowledged that "society's accumulated myths and fears about disability are as handicapping as are the physical limitations that flow from actual impairment."[33] Regulations and courts addressing job discrimination, based on disability under the ADA and other laws, have expressly identified the discrimination that results from misperceptions and unrealistically low expectations of what people with disabilities are able to do.[34] One legal commentator has written that "[t]he image of a [person with a disability] as one who is not able to do many things, who is unable to fill a proper role in society, and who is not a success in terms of achievements or happiness is widespread and deep-seated."[35]

In reality, such attitudes and negative predictions of life quality have little to do with the actual life experiences of people with disabilities. People with disabilities commonly report more satisfaction with their lives than others might have expected. Though they commonly encounter obstacles, prejudice, and discrimination, most people with disabilities manage to derive satisfaction and pleasure from their lives. After conducting a nationwide poll of people with disabilities, Louis Harris and Associates reported that "[d]espite their disadvantaged status and frequent exclusion from activities enjoyed by most Americans, a large majority of disabled Americans are satisfied with their lives"; the Harris organization described this as "a remarkable finding in light of the portrait of hardships revealed in these survey findings."[36] Even individuals who identified themselves as having very severe disabilities tended to report that they were very or somewhat satisfied with their lives.[37]

Nor do disabilities generally have the devastating effect upon the social milestones of marriage and having children that some might expect. There is virtually no difference between the proportion of Americans with disabilities and those without who are married,[38] and most people with disabilities do not consider their disability to have much impact on their ability to have children or their interest in doing so.[39] Even people with severe pain and highly invasive medical treatments report higher life satisfaction than others expect.[40]

The realities of the quality of the lives of Americans with disabilities is obscured by the misguided projections and low expectations of others, for as one disability authority has observed, "When society opts to judge the quality of life for an individual with a disability, it does so from the perspective of a fear of disability and historical prejudice and discrimination."[41]

5. Fallibility of medical predictions

Many people with disabilities have been great beneficiaries of the miracles of modern medicine. Some owe their very lives, and others much of their ability to function, to the medical profession. Lifesaving treatments, rehabilitative surgical techniques, new medications, and numerous other medical advances have greatly improved chances for survival, the amelioration of limitations, and options for accommodating disabilities. And yet people with disabilities have also frequently seen firsthand evidence that medicine is not totally a science but still something of an art, particularly in regard to the imperfections of medical prognosticating. Individuals with disabilities and parents of children with disabilities have encountered numerous kinds of fervently pronounced, but inaccurate predictions by members of the medical professional. Some have been told that they or their children would not survive, or would not regain consciousness, or would not walk, or would not read, or would not be toilet-trained, or could not live independently, or could not perform particular activities, and yet ultimately found these predictions to be wildly inaccurate. Other people have been confined and subjected to involuntary treatment regimes, based upon notoriously unreliable predictions about their supposed proclivities, ability to cope, or even dangerousness, based upon the application of psychiatric labels.

Predictions of patients' life expectancy are particularly difficult and unreliable.[42] Indeed, "[a] surprising number of people have had the experience of being misinformed that they had a terminal illness."[43] Evan Kemp, former chairman of the Equal Employment Opportunity Commission, who was diagnosed with a progressive neuromuscular disease at age 12, has written:

> *"Upon diagnosis, my parents were informed by the physicians treating me that I would die within two years. Later, another group of physicians was certain that I would live only to the age of 18. Yet here I am at age 59, continuing to have an extraordinarily high quality of life… And my case is by no means unique. The majority of families I have encountered in my lifetime, and who have been close enough to share details of their extended family life, have had at least one member who defied the medical establishment by living a far longer and more productive life than expected."*[44]

One noteworthy example of erroneous medical predicting grew out of an early, widely publicized court case[45] in which permission was sought to discontinue a ventilator for a comatose young woman named Karen Quinlan. There was no dispute among the medical experts that without the assistance of the ventilator, Ms. Quinlan would die in a matter of days or weeks, if not hours. After the New Jersey courts approved discontinuance of the ventilator, it was removed, but Karen Quinlan stayed alive, breathing on her own, for almost ten years. However one feels about the court's decision in the Quinlan matter, it is clear that the medical forecasting was substantially erroneous in this highly visible, carefully considered, fully litigated situation. This is not to suggest that most, or even a substantial portion, of medical forecasting is erroneous, but people with disabilities are aware of enough instances of dramatic mistakes that many of them have a healthy skepticism of medical predictions, particularly as it relates to future life quality. Medical personnel are generally not very knowledgeable of special education and rehabilitation techniques, specialized accommodations, independent-living philosophy, and other factors that may spell the difference between a direly limited or a satisfying and fulfilling future for an individual with a disability.

6. Eschewing the Medical Model of Disabilities

In its *Achieving Independence* report, the Council observed that a "disability rights perspective…stands in contrast to a medical model, which views people with disabilities as needing to be cured."[46] The medical model imposes certain expectations upon both the medical personnel and the "patient."[47] It places primary responsibility for diagnosis and treatment in the hands of medical practitioners. Physicians are deemed to be the technically competent experts for addressing the patient's needs through an established chain of command to other medical personnel. The patients, for their part, are expected to play the roles of "sick" or "impaired" persons; this entails an exemption from some ordinary social activities and responsibilities, and an expectation that they will cooperate with the attending medical practitioners in "getting well".[48] The medical model views people with disabilities as "victims" of a medical problem in need of treatment, not as responsible adults in need of rights and respect.[49]

People with disabilities have first-hand experience with the medical model in various service delivery systems including hospitals and some rehabilitation facilities, and sometimes, often in its most egregious form, in mental health treatment facilities. The application of the medical model in the mental health context has been widely described and vehemently criticized by various commentators.[50] Frequently, it has involved the involuntary institutionalization of individuals based upon a dubious psychiatric diagnosis, enforced confinement on locked wards in a control-oriented regime, with limited freedoms conditioned upon compliance with the rules of the facility, as well as "treatment" which may be unwanted, most frequently, the administration of powerful psychotropic drugs or controversial electroshock "therapy". As commentators have noted: "First and foremost, programs reflect the medical-model mentality that perceives people with mental disabilities as perpetual patients, with the resultant infantilization that so often accompanies that status."[51]

Many people with disabilities reject the behavioral expectations imposed upon them by such roles, and "do not want to be relieved of their familial, occupational, and civic responsibilities in exchange for a childlike dependency."[52] Clearly the medical model is contrary to the notions of independent living, consumer self-direction, and freedom of choice discussed in section 3 above. From an independent living perspective:

> *The pathology is not in the individual, as the medical model would suggest, but rather in the physical, social, political and economic environment that has up to now limited the choices available to people with disabilities. The solution to these problems is not more professional intervention but more self-help initiatives leading to the removal of barriers and to the full participation of disabled people in society.*[53]

Again, this is not to suggest that people with disabilities have not received great benefits from various medical interventions, assuming truly informed consent has been obtained — from treatments and therapies provided by medical personnel and from the treatment techniques, devices, and medications available at modern medical facilities. Nonetheless, many people with disabilities view the medical model as a poor prism, for themselves and our society, through which to view the reality of their lives with disabilities.

7. The impact of onset of disability upon emotional state and decision-making

When a person is not born with a disability, the onset of a substantially impairing condition and the awareness of one's new physical or mental limitations usually come as a blow to a person's self-image and psychological balance. Disabilities that are the result of violence, accident, or illness usually are accompanied by additional emotional repercussions. The inception of disabilities is often associated with a period of hospitalization or other intense medical intervention that adds additional disorientation.

Pain and medication may take an additional toll on emotional equilibrium. Family members and friends may be devastated by what has happened and find it hard to relate to the individual in ways they normally did in the past. Neither the individual with the new disability nor friends and family members may have any idea how people adapt to such a condition, any concept of rehabilitation possibilities, nor a clue that many people are living fulfilling and joyful lives with the same or even more severe conditions. To a person newly confronted with the realization that he or she has a disability, it may appear that the "whole world has been turned upside down." Strong feelings of fear, helplessness, anger, sadness, shame, and confusion are common.

It is typical, therefore, for people who have recently been confronted with a disability to experience a period of disorientation and depression. With proper assistance and information, such disorientation and depression usually abate over time. It may follow a pattern of denial, anger, hopelessness, adjustment that characterize the grieving process for various kinds of serious losses. Sometimes medication, psychotherapy, or other treatment may be necessary to help deal with lingering depression. Most people with disabilities gradually come to accept and live constructively with their disabilities. They may undergo rehabilitation and learn techniques for adapting to and surmounting limitations; they may discover that there are devices and accommodations that will make them more independent, productive, and comfortable; they may find that many other people have similar conditions and are managing to do quite well anyway. Generally, the feelings of helplessness and sadness fade away to a manageable level over time.

The existence of a normal period of disorientation and depression following the acquisition of a disability makes it imperative that people in such a situation not try to make long-term or irreversible decisions that may be colored by the temporary depression and disorientation rather than by an exercise of sound judgment. Medical personnel cannot be counted on to distinguish between the two situations, for "physicians responding to requests for assistance are often inadequately trained to distinguish rational requests from those driven by depression."[54] The experience of numerous people with disabilities is that they would have been unable to make truly rational decisions while still in the throes of the unsettled state of mind that commonly accompanies the onset of a disabling condition. Moreover, during such a period of confusion and emotional instability, people are particularly vulnerable to duress, intimidation, and coercion by those around them.

In addition, people newly confronted with a disability "may have internalized society's prejudices against persons with disabilities or developed fears about living with a disability. With counseling and time, however, such notions or feelings can dissipate."[55] With proper information, support, and care, the depths of disorientation and overwhelming sadness will usually ease with the passage of time and the person with a new disability will have a chance to integrate the idea of having a disability, to learn ways to manage it and its consequences, and to return to the quest confronting all human beings of trying to wrest a reasonable degree of happiness and fulfillment from our existence.

8. The reality of living with pain and bodily malfunction

Some individuals with disabilities have had to confront severe pain, sometimes chronic pain, and have experienced the two-edged reality of living with such pain. On the one hand, they have encountered the truly debilitating effects of chronic pain that saps one's strength and drains one's psyche. Only persons who have experienced significant, long-term pain fully understand its crushing impact. On the other hand, many people have learned firsthand that there are a variety of techniques for treating pain, including various medications, biofeedback, nerve treatments, hypnosis, and other nonobtrusive alternative medical treatments. Moreover, even in the rarer situations where pain is essentially untreatable, some individuals have learned to successfully live with their pain, and report life satisfaction and desire to continue living, despite their pain.[56]

From these varying experiences, one learns that some people's pain can be treated and ameliorated, others can learn to manage and live with their pain, and still others experience pain that cannot be eased and that they find themselves unable to endure. The very real impact of chronic, severe, untreatable pain should not be underestimated.

People with disabilities also have considerable experience in dealing with the malfunctioning, breakdown, or absence of normal body parts or mental processes. Having learned to deal with such imperfect functioning as part of their ongoing day-to-day existence, people with disabilities are much less likely to be horrified by such physical or mental dysfunction. Consequently, people with disabilities tend to be much more aware than the general public that one can lead a valid, happy life even though one's legs, or eyes, or arms, or memory, or bladder, or ears, or mouth, or brain, or genitals, or sensory processing, or hands, or whatever other parts of the body or mind are not working properly.

A key implication of people-with-disabilities' experience with pain and dysfunction is the need for more frequent and informed use of pain relief medication. The American Medical Association (AMA) and the United States Government have both acknowledged that physicians have not done an adequate job in treating pain.[57] To address this problem, the AMA, the

American Board of Internal Medicine, the American Academy of Hospice and Palliative Medicine, and other medical organization have undertaken various initiatives to improve the training and continuing education of doctors in pain-relief measures for persons with terminal medical conditions.[58] According to medical authorities, many physicians are not sufficiently familiar with the use of various treatments, including heavy doses of morphine, to control pain in dying patients.[59]

Medical ethics standards permit doctors to prescribe medication to relieve pain even if the necessary dose will hasten death.[60] Better training of physicians in techniques and standards for treatment of pain should be a primary goal, so that all individuals who are confronted with serious pain can have maximum relief. Moreover, hospice and other programs and treatments to make the process of dying more comfortable and peaceful should be made widely available.

9. Divergent Interests of Those Involved in Assisted-Suicide Decisions

As they have undertaken to attain independence and self-determination in their lives — to make the kinds of choices regarding their own activities, living arrangements, and means for pursuing happiness that other Americans take for granted — citizens with disabilities have become sharply aware of the fact that their interests often diverge from those of others who would seek to act "in their best interest." Medical personnel, officials of residential and other care-giving facilities, religious officials, social workers, rehabilitation professionals, and even family members often have views as to what would be best for an individual with a disability that are drastically different from what she or he actually wants. This becomes particularly true when there may be other interests or agendas being pursued by these other parties.

Decisions about medical care are particularly subject to such separate, and often conflicting, interests in the outcome. Physicians may have concerns about prolonging treatment of patients whom they are unable to "cure", and psychological pain about continuing to see patients for whom they have "failed." Or they may have pressures from too heavy a patient load. Overcrowded medical facilities may need "the bed" that the patient is occupying. The doctor and the medical facility may be concerned about insurance limits on extended treatment, or the exhaustion of financial resources of the patient or the patient's family, and fear that the bill for continued care will never be paid. Conferring medical peers may have various motivations including mutual back-scratching, professional deference, or career goals that render peer review a mere rubberstamping. Other medical personnel and related professionals may have their own personal or philosophical axes to grind.

Family members may have any number of tensions, disputes, agendas, and pressures, not the least of which may be financial concerns, or emotional strain or exhaustion from the ordeal of extended medical treatment of a family member, or of having a close relative diagnosed with a terminal condition. In what hopefully are rarer cases, a close relative may have actual animosity toward the person who is undergoing treatment or may be involved in a love triangle or some other conflict-filled situation. People with disabilities would generally be unwilling to let doctors, nurses, medical-review panels, or their own families make judgments in their place concerning something as important as their health and very life.

V. Conclusions

Based upon the foregoing insights derived from the experience of people with disabilities and the existing legal framework, the National Council on Disability has grappled to arrive at a constructive, principled position on the issue of physician-assisted suicide for persons with imminently terminal conditions. To some degree, this effort has appeared to be like the plight of the mythical Jason whose ship, the Argo, had to sail between the two monsters, Charybdis and Scylla — neither choice is very appealing.

Opposing the legalization of assisted suicide seemingly deprives people with disabilities faced with imminent death and severe pain, the only power they can have to decide when and how they will die, an ability to choose that might offer them some control, dignity, and measure of self-determination in an otherwise bleak situation; such control of one's own destiny, freedom of choice, and self-determination are key principles of the disability rights and independent-living philosophies and cornerstones of the initiatives which the Council has advocated.

On the other hand, legalizing assisted suicide seems to risk its likely use, the ultimate manifestation of prejudice against people with disabilities in our society, as a means to unnecessarily end, or to coerce the end, of people with disabilities' lives; persons with disabilities know that many in society believe that they would be better off dead, and legalized assisted suicide offers a subtle and sometimes not-so-subtle way to make that judgment a reality.

To resolve this dilemma, the Council has weighed the pros and cons very carefully. Among other considerations, it has found the following to weigh very heavily in its deliberations:

The current situation

Under current law, most people who choose to commit suicide can do so without the assistance of a physician. Only a small number of people having disabilities are unable to terminate their lives if they choose to do so. Patients have the right to refuse medical treatments, even lifesaving or life-prolonging measures; informed consent of the patient is a legal prerequisite for the initiation or continuation of medical treatment. Physicians are permitted under current medical standards to prescribe medication as necessary to control pain, even if the necessary dosage will result in hastening the patient's death. Most, though not all, pain, even if severe, can be controlled by the proper administration of medication; better training of physicians would improve effective treatment of pain. Many individuals learn to live satisfying lives in spite of experiencing severe pain.

People with disabilities' lives are frequently viewed as valueless by others, including members of the medical profession. People with disabilities are often harassed and coerced to end their lives when faced with life-threatening conditions, even if the conditions are imminently treatable; others have had their lives involuntarily terminated by medical personnel. These practices manifest blatant prejudice and are a virulent form of the discrimination that the Americans with Disabilities Act, and other laws, condemn. Legal and medical authorities should denounce and prohibit any attempt to pressure, harass, or coerce any individual to shorten her or his life; they should certainly proscribe any action to terminate an individual's life, taken without that person's full, voluntary, and informed consent, whether it be called "suicide," "mercy killing," "letting nature take its course," or some other euphemistic term. And certainly there should be official condemnation and cessation of practices by which people with disabilities are pressured to sign "Do-Not-Resuscitate" consent forms; or such forms are hidden within a stack of admission and consent papers, in the hope that the individual with a disability will sign them without paying attention to what is being signed.

Procedural protections

As a potential escape hatch from the dilemma described above, the Council considered the possibility that a properly devised set of procedural protections could permit physician-assisted suicide to occur in limited circumstances while preventing it from being abused or applied improperly to the disadvantage of people with disabilities. There have been various proposals of such procedural safeguards or the elements they should contain.[61] An article in the *New England Journal of Medicine* proposed a system in which treating physicians would be prohibited from complying with a patient's request for assisted suicide unless the request was approved by a physician "palliative care specialist" and by a "regional palliative care committee" with both lay and professional members.[62] In the Netherlands, assisted suicides (and active euthanasia) are permitted by the courts if they satisfy nine criteria that impose a combination of substantive platitudes and procedural standards:

1. The patient must be suffering unbearably;
2. The patient must be conscious when he expresses the desire to die;
3. The request for euthanasia must be voluntary;
4. The patient must have been given alternatives with time to consider them;
5. There must be viable solutions for the patient;
6. The death must not inflict unnecessary suffering on others;

7. The decision must involve more than one person;

8. Only a physician may perform the euthanasia; and

9. The physician must exercise great care in making the decision.[63]

These limited procedural protections have certainly not worked. As Representative Charles Canady, Chair of the Subcommittee on the Constitution of the U.S. House of Representatives has reported, the Netherlands procedures "give an enormous amount of discretion to doctors, and, consequently, give very little protection to patients."[64] As a result, non-voluntary euthanasia is being widely performed in the Netherlands.[65]

One of the briefs filed in favor of legalizing physician-assisted suicide in the pending Supreme Court cases suggested that states might impose the following safeguards:

- Requiring the individual to repeat the request on more than one occasion;
- Requiring the request to be made to more than one doctor;
- Requiring the individual to be provided an opportunity to discuss the problem with a mental health professional;
- Requiring the individual to be informed of programs and resources that are available to improve the quality of his or her remaining life; and
- Requiring the individual to be informed on several occasions that he or she may, and is encouraged to, change his/her mind at any time.[66]

The vigorous implementation of these various proposals would still fall far short of protecting the rights and interests of people with disabilities. To effectively limit assisted suicides to appropriate situations and make certain that they do not become a vehicle for fatal discrimination against people with disabilities, such procedures would, at a minimum, have to ensure: that the patient's diagnosis is completely accurate; that the condition of the patient is definitely terminal; that the patient's death is imminent; that there are no available treatments that can save or significantly prolong the patient's life; that the patient is suffering unendurable pain and this pain cannot be controlled by medication or alternative treatments or therapies; that the patient wishes to commit suicide; that the patient's decision is based upon full information about the patient's diagnosis, prognosis, and options, and the patient has understood this information; that the patient's desire to die is not a result of temporary dejection resulting from disorientation, adjusting to new limitations, or other causes; that the patient's desire to die is not a result of prejudice, stereotypes, and misinformation about people with disabilities and living with a disability; that the patient's decision to seek suicide is reached only after the patient has received, from knowledgeable, disinterested sources, a thorough exploration and explanation of treatment options, rehabilitative techniques, assistive devices, accommodations, etc., for living successfully with the patient's disabilities; that the patient has had the opportunity to meet and talk at length with people living with similar disabilities; that the patient has made the decision to choose suicide freely without being influenced by coercion, harassment, intimidation, or duress; that the patient has requested physician-assisted suicide repeatedly over a sufficiently long period of time to ensure that it represents a determined steady conviction to end his or her life; that the patient is unable to commit suicide without the assistance of a physician; and that there is oversight by responsible, objective, disinterested, and impartial authorities who can verify whether or not the foregoing prerequisites to a patient's decision to choose suicide have been satisfied.

It may be possible to construct procedural safeguards to ensure that some of these elements are fulfilled in particular circumstances. Given the current state of medical science and human institutions, however, it may be nearly impossible for some of these prerequisites to be satisfied. The diagnosis that conditions are terminal and that death is imminent are not totally reliable. Relative assessments of pain and the state of mind or motivation of patients are not objectively measurable and thus are hard to verify. Medical personnel with an agenda of promoting assisted suicide may influence patients and manipulate the procedural safeguards. Individuals who are hospitalized, medicated, and faced with a serious health problem are very vulnerable to subtle psychological pressures from their care providers and loved ones. Medical reviews and second opinions are subject to professional deference and conflicts of interest. Can medical authorities realistically attest that the patient has received adequate information about resources, accommodations, assistive devices, and other matters enhancing one's option in living with a disability?

More importantly, however, the more stringent and encompassing one seeks to make procedural safeguards in this context, the more intrusive they become, and the greater the extent to which doctors and psychiatrists become the gatekeepers. Putting the procedures in a judicial or quasi-judicial setting would not avoid this problem, because most of the testimony and opinions would still have to come from medical practitioners, consultants, and experts; the medical profession would still serve as gatekeepers, but now there would be lawyers and judges involved, too, as overseers. Establishing with certainty that a particular patient has the mental competence and emotional balance for making the decision to die will inevitably involve psychiatric evaluations. As the procedural noose tightens to prevent erroneous and inappropriate assisted suicides, the individual's privacy and control of the situation fly out the window, and the medical model runs rampant. Ironically, the pursuit of assisted suicide in the name of individual liberty would wind up necessitating egregious restrictions and highly invasive participation by members of the medical and legal professions.

Weighing the dangers of physician-assisted suicide against its benefits

The benefits of permitting physician-assisted suicide have been ably argued by advocates of its legalization. They include respect for individual autonomy, liberty, and the right to make one's own choices about matters concerning one's intimate personal welfare; affording the dignity of control and choice for a patient who otherwise has little control of her or his situation; allowing the patient to select the time and circumstances of death, rather than being totally at the mercy of the terminal medical condition; safeguarding the doctor/patient relationship in making this final medical decision; giving the patient the option of dying in an alert condition rather than in a medicated haze during the last hours of life; and, most importantly, giving the patient the ability to avoid severe pain and suffering. Some of these benefits for the individuals involved are substantial and should not be discounted.

Whatever beneficial consequences of physician-assisted suicide there may be, however, the benefits only apply to the small number of people who actually have an imminently terminal condition, are in severe, untreatable pain, wish to commit suicide, and are unable to do so by themselves. Many terminal patients enduring pain do not wish to terminate their lives.[67] Most of those who do can, do so without a doctor's involvement.

The dangers of permitting physician-assisted suicide are large indeed. The pressures upon people with disabilities to choose to end their lives, and the insidious appropriation by others of the right to make that choice for them are already way too common in our society. These pressures are increasing and will continue to grow as managed health care and limitations upon health care resources precipitate increased "rationing" of health care services and health care financing.[68]

There is no doubt that people with disabilities are among society's most likely candidates for ending their lives. As the experience in the Netherlands demonstrates,[69] there is also little doubt that legalizing assisted suicide generates strong pressures upon individuals and families to utilize that option, and leads very quickly to coercion and involuntary euthanasia. The so-called "slippery slope" already operates in regard to individuals with disabilities and decisions to discontinue life-support systems and "Do-Not-Resuscitate" orders; it would expand dramatically if physician-assisted suicide were to become legal. Moreover, not only would the lives of people with any disability deemed too difficult to live with be at risk, but persons with disabilities who are poor or members of racial minorities are likely to be in the most jeopardy of all.

If assisted suicide were to be legalized, the most dire ramifications for people with disabilities would ensue unless stringent procedural prerequisites were established to prevent its misuse, abuse, improper application, and creeping expansion. But, to be effective, such procedural safeguards would necessarily sacrifice individual autonomy to the supervision of medical and legal overlords to an unacceptable degree — the cure in this case being as bad as the disease.

At its core, legalization of physician-assisted suicide would represent a recognition by society that some particular individuals have gotten all the substantial positive benefits they are going to get from their lives, and, in the face of serious pain and suffering they would endure if they continue to live, the few more hours or days they can wring out of existence are not worth it; for such individuals society would be saying that death is preferable to life, and physicians would be empowered to help them terminate their lives. For many people with disabilities, society has frequently made it clear that it believes they would be better off dead, or better that they had not been born. But it is more often the discrimination, prejudice, and barriers that they encounter, and the restrictions and lack of options that this society has imposed, rather than their disabilities or their physical pain, that cause people with disabilities' lives to be unsatisfactory and painful.

In proposals to legalize assisted suicide, proponents are sometimes willing to agree that a decision to choose suicide must be preceded by a full explanation of the programs, resources, and options available to assist the patient if he or she does not decide to pursue suicide.[70] Many people with disabilities find this to be a very shallow promise when they know that all too often the programs are too few, the resources are too limited, and the options, very often, are nonexistent. Society should not be ready to give up on the lives of its citizens with disabilities until it has made real and persistent efforts to give these citizens a fair and equal chance to achieve a meaningful life.[71] Some of the energy being devoted to promoting assisted suicide might be put to better use in helping to improve the lives of people with disabilities.

For all of these reasons, the Council has decided that at this time in the history of American society, it opposes the legalization of assisted suicide. Current evidence indicates clearly that the interests of the few people who would benefit from legalizing physician-assisted suicide are heavily outweighed by the probability that any law, procedures, and standards that can be imposed to regulate physician-assisted suicide will be misapplied to unnecessarily end the lives of people with disabilities, and entail an intolerable degree of intervention by legal and medical officials in such decisions. On balance, the current illegality of physician-assisted suicide is preferable to the limited benefits to be gained by its legalization. At least until such time as our society provides a comprehensive, fully funded, and operational system of assistive-living services for people with disabilities, this is the only position that the National Council on Disability can, in good conscience, support.

References

1. David Orentlicher, M.D., J.D., The legalization of physician assisted suicide, *New England Journal of Medicine* 335: 663, 665 (Aug. 29, 1996).
2. No. 95-1858, October Term, 1996.
3. No. 96-110, October Term, 1996.
4. 497 U.S. 261 (1990).

5. No. 95-1858, October Term, 1996.
6. *Quill v. Vacco*, 80 F 3d 716 (2d Cir 1996).
7. *Id.*, 729.
8. No. 96-110, October Term, 1996.
9. National Hospice Association, *Hospice in Brief* at p. 1.
10. *Id.*
11. National Hospice Association, *Hospice Fact Sheet* at p. 1 (Jan. 1, 1997).
12. *Id.*, p. 2, citing a 1995 study by Lewin-VHI and a 1988 study conducted by the Health Care Financing Administration (HCFA).
13. For a good overview and additional information about hospice programs, *see, e.g.*, Larry Beresford, *The Hospice Handbook* (1993).
14. *Report of the United Nations Expert Group Meeting on Barrier-Free Design*, 26 Int. Rehab. Review 3 (1975).
15. *State v. McAfee*, 385 S E 2d 651 (GA 1989).
16. *McKay v. Bergstedt*, 801 P 2d 617, 624-35 (NV 1990).
17. *Id.*, 637.
18. *Id.*, 628.
19. 42 U.S.C. §12101(a)(2).
20. *Id.*, §12101(a)(7).
21. *Id.*, §12101(a)(2).
22. U.S. Commn on Civil Rights, *Accommodating the Spectrum of Individual Abilities* 35-36 (1983).
23. *See, e.g., Accommodating the Spectrum of Individual Abilities* 17-42, 159; *Alexander v. Choate*, 469 U.S. 287, 295-96, 286 (quoting 117 Cong. Rec. 45,974 (1971) (statement of Rep. Vanik); 118 Cong. Rec. 526 (1972) (statement of Sen. Percy)) (1985); S. Rep. No. 116, 101st Cong., 1st Sess. 9 (1989); H.R. Rep. No. 485, 101st Cong., 2d Sess. pt. 2, at 32 (1990) (Education and Labor Committee) [hereinafter *Education & Labor Committee Report*]; *Task Force on the Rights & Empowerment of Americans with Disabilities, Equality for 43 Million Americans with Disabilities: A Moral and Economic Imperative* 8 (1990), quoted in *Education & Labor Committee Report*, at 31-32; Louis Harris & Assocs., *The ICD Survey of Disabled Americans: Bringing Disabled Americans into the Mainstream* 70, 75 (1986); Louis Harris & Assocs., *The ICD Survey II: Employing Disabled Americans* 12 (1987); *City of Cleburne v. Cleburne Living Center*, 473 U.S. 432, 454 (Stevens, J., joined by Burger, C.J., concurring) (1985); *id.*, 461, 462 (Marshall, J., joined by Brennan & Blackmun, JJ., concurring in part and dissenting in part).
24. *See, e.g.*, 29 U.S.C. §§ 701(a)&(b), 706(20), 706(30), 796a(1), 796d(a), 796c(a)(2); 42 U.S.C. §§ 8013(4), 12101(a)(8).
25. *Accommodating the Spectrum, supra* n. 17, at 83-84, quoting Timothy M. Cole, "What's new about independent living?," 60 *Archives Physical Med. & Rehabilitation* 458-62 (1979)).
26. Center for Independent Living, Independent living: the right to choose, in *Disabled People as Second-Class Citizens* 248 (Eisenberg, Griggins, & Duval eds., 1982) (quoted in *Accommodating the Spectrum, supra* n. 17, at 84).
27. Gini Laurie, Independent living programs, 22 *Rehabilitation Gazette* 9-11 (1979) (quoted in *Accommodating the Spectrum, supra* n. 17, at 83).

28. *See, e.g., Accommodating the Spectrum, supra* n. 17, at 85, and authorities cited therein.

29. Gerben DeJong, Independent living: from social movement to analytic paradigm, 60 *Archives Physical Med. & Rehabilitation* 435-46 (1979) (quoted in *Accommodating the Spectrum, supra* n. 17, at 85).

30. *Id.*, §701(a)(3), *as amended by* Pub. L. No. 102-569, tit. I, §101, 106 Stat. 4346 (1992).

31. *Id.*, §701(a)(6), *as amended by* Pub. L. No. 102-569, tit. I, §101, 106 Stat. 4346 (1992).

32. U.S. Commn on Civil Rights, *Accommodating the Spectrum of Individual Abilities* 26 (1983)

33. *School Board of Nassau County v. Arline*, 480 US 273, 284-85 (1987).

34. 29 C.F.R. 406 (app. to pt. 1630) (commentary on §1630.2(l)) (1993) (can prove discrimination "by demonstrating that the exclusion was caused by one of the 'common attitudinal barriers' toward individuals with disabilities such as an employer's concern about productivity, safety, insurance, liability, attendance, cost of accommodation and accessibility, workers compensation costs, and acceptance by co-workers and customers"); *Wooten v. Farmland Foods*, 58 F 3d 382, 385 (8th Cir 1995) (the "regarded as" prong of the definition of disability encompasses "archaic attitudes, erroneous perceptions, and myths"). Several ADA decisions have recognized employers' "myths, fears and stereotypes associated with disabilities." *See, e.g., Freund v. Lockheed Missiles and Space Co.*, 930 F.Supp. 613, 618 (S.D.Ga. 1996); *EEOC v. Texas Bus Lines*, 923 F.Supp. 965, 975 (S.D.Tex. 1996); *Howard v. Navistar Internat'l Transp. Corp.*, 904 F.Supp. 922, 929-30 (E.D.Wis. 1995); *Pritchard v. Southern Company Services*, 1995 WL 338662, 4 AD Cases 465, 473 (N.D.Ala. 1995); *Lussier v. Runyon*, 1994 WL 129776, 3 AD Cases 223, 231 (D.Me. 1994); *Scharff v. Frank*, 791 F.Supp. 182, 187 (S.D.Oh. 1991) ("stereotypical treatment").

35. Robert L. Burgdorf Jr., *The Legal Rights of Handicapped Persons: Cases, Materials, and Text* 8 (1980).

36. Louis Harris & Assocs., *The ICD Survey of Disabled Americans: Bringing Disabled Americans into the Mainstream* 55 (1986).

37. *Id.*, 46, Table 19.

38. *Id.*, 42.

39. *Id.*, 42 (only 7% of persons with disabilities say that their disability has a negative effect on their ability to, or interest in, having children).

40. *See, e.g.*, J.R. Bach & M.C. Tilton, Life satisfaction and well-being measures in ventilator-assisted individuals with traumatic tetraplegia, 75 *Arch. of Physical Med. & Rehab.* 626 (1994).

41. Paul Steven Miller, The impact of assisted suicide on persons with disabilities — is it a right without freedom?, *Issues in Law & Medicine* 9:47, 54 (1993).

42. *See, e.g.*, Joanne Lynn, et al., *Accurate Prognostications of Death: Opportunities and Challenges for Clinicians*, 163 W.J.Med. 250, 251 (1995).

43. Richard A. Posner, *Aging and Old Age* 245 (1995).

44. Evan J. Kemp, Jr., Could you please die now?: disabled people like me have good reason to fear the push for assisted suicide, *The Washington Post* C1 (Jan. 5, 1997).

45. In re Quinlan, 355 A.2d 647 (N.J. 1976).
46. National Council on Disability, *Achieving Independence: The Challenge for the 21st Century* 19 (1996).
47. *See, e.g.*, Gerben DeJong, *Independent Living: From Social Movement to Analytic Paradigm*, 39, 50-51 (Robert P. Marinelli & Arthur E. Dell Orto, eds., 1984).
48. *Id.*, 52-53.
49. Douglas Biklen, The myth of clinical judgment, *Journal of Social Issues* Vol. 44: 127, 128 (1988).
50. *See, e.g.*, Erving Goffman. *Asylums: Essays on the Social Situation of Mental Patients and Other Inmates.* Garden City, N.J.: Anchor Books; Thomas S. Szasz. 1961. *The Myth of Mental Illness.* New York: Harper and Row; Thomas S. Szasz. 1970. *The Manufacture of Madness: A Comparative Study of the Inquisition and the Mental Health Movement.* New York: Dell; R.D. Laing. 1967. *The Politics of Experience.* New York: Pantheon Press; Ethan Fromm. 1970. *The Crisis of Psychoanalysis.* New York: Holt, Rinehart and Winston; E. Fuller Torrey. 1975. *The Death of Psychiatry.* New York: Penguin Books; John Gliedman & William Roth. 1980. *The Unexpected Minority: Handicapped Children in America.* New York: Harcourt Brace Jovanovich; Bonnie Milstein & Steven Hitov. 1993. Housing and the ADA. In Lawrence O. Gostin & Henry A. Beyer, eds. *Implementing the Americans with Disabilities Act: Rights and Responsibilities of All Americans*, 137, 144-47. Baltimore, MD: Paul H. Brookes Publishing Co.
51. Bonnie Milstein & Steven Hitov. 1993. Housing and the ADA. In Lawrence O. Gostin & Henry A. Beyer, eds. *Implementing the Americans with Disabilities Act: Rights and Responsibilities of All Americans*, 137, 145-46. Baltimore, MD: Paul H. Brookes Publishing Co.
52. DeJong, *supra*, at 52.
53. Gerben DeJong and Raymond Lifchez, Physical disability and public policy, *The Scientific American* 248: 41, 45 (1983).
54. David Orentlicher, M.D., J.D., The legalization of physician-assisted suicide, *New England Journal of Medicine* 335: 663, 664 (Aug. 29, 1996), citing Y. Conwell & E.D. Caine, Rational suicide and the right to die—reality and myth," *New England Journal of Medicine* 325: 1100-03 (1991).
55. Paul Steven Miller, The impact of assisted suicide on persons with disabilities—is it a right without freedom?, *Issues in Law & Medicine* 9:47, 58 (1993).
56. *See, e.g.*, J.R. Bach & M.C. Tilton, Life satisfaction and well-being measures in ventilator-assisted individuals with traumatic tetraplegia, 75 *Arch. of Physical Med. & Rehab.* 626 (1994); Ezekiel J. Emmanuel, Diane L. Fairclough, Elisabeth R. Daniel, & Brian R. Clarridge, Euthanasia: physician assisted suicide: attitude and experiences of oncology patients, oncologists, and the public, *Lancet* 347: 1805-10 (1996).
57. Knight Ridder/Tribune, AMA to teach doctors to aid the dying, *Chicago Tribune* p. 1A10 (Dec. 13, 1996); Brief for the United States as Amicus Curiae Supporting Petitioners in *Vacco v. Quill*, No. 95-1858, October Term, 1996 at p. 9 (referring to "health care system that often undertreats patients' pain"); Brief for the United States as Amicus Curiae Supporting Petitioners in *State of Washington v. Glucksberg*, No. 96-110, October Term, 1996, at p. 19 ("inadequately treated pain").

58. Knight Ridder/Tribune, AMA to teach doctors to aid the dying, *Chicago Tribune* p. 1A10 (Dec. 13, 1996).

59. *Id.*

60. AMA Council on Ethical and Judicial Affairs, *Code of Medical Ethics: Current Opinions* § 2.20 (1989), *cited in* Brief for the United States as Amicus Curiae Supporting Petitioners in *State of Washington v. Glucksberg*, No. 96-110, October Term, 1996, at p. 17.

61. In the related context of discontinuance of life-prolonging treatment for patients totally unable to make the decisions themselves, some courts have required various procedural safeguards. See *Superintendent of Belchertown v. Saikewicz*, 370 N.E.2d 417 (Mass. 1977) (required approval in court proceeding with appointment of a guardian ad litem to represent the interests of the patient); In re Quinlan, 355 A.2d 647 (N.J. 1976) (required combined agreement of the attending doctors, the family, and hospital review panel).

62. Franklin G. Miller, Timothy E. Quill, Howard Brody, John G. Fletcher, Lawrence O. Gostin, & Diane E. Meier, Regulating physician-assisted death, *The New England Journal of Medicine* 331: 119-122 (July 14, 1994).

63. *Report of Chairman Charles T. Canady to the Subcommittee on the Constitution of the Committee on the Judiciary of the House of Representatives* 104 Cong., 2d Sess., p. 6 (September 1996). In 1986, the Royal Dutch Medical Association published *Guidelines for Euthanasia,* which establishes five criteria: "voluntariness," "a well considered request," "persistent desire for death," "unacceptable suffering," and "collegial consultation." *Id.* at 8, quoting Jürgen Wöretshofer & Matthias Borgers, The Dutch procedure for mercy killing and assisted suicide by physicians in a national and international perspective," *Maastricht Journal of European and Comparative Law* 2:2, 7 (1996).

64. *Report of Chairman Charles T. Canady to the Subcommittee on the Constitution of the Committee on the Judiciary of the House of Representatives* 104 Cong., 2d Sess., p. 11 (September 1996).

65. *Id.,* p. 1.

66. Brief for Amici Curiae, Gay Men's Health Crisis *et al.* in *Vacco v. Quill,* No. 95-1858, and *State of Washington v. Glucksberg,* No. 96-110, October Term, 1996, at p. 15.

67. *See, e.g.,* Ezekiel J. Emmanuel, Diane L. Fairclough, Elisabeth R. Daniel, & Brian R. Clarridge, Euthanasia: physician-assisted suicide: attitude and experiences of oncology patients, oncologists, and the public, *Lancet* 347: 1805-10 (1996) (cancer patients enduring pain not inclined to want euthanasia or assisted suicide).

68. One author has observed that, as health care costs increase, while funding for health care and supportive programs is restricted, "assisted suicide becomes a more cost-effective, expedient, and ultimately socially acceptable option." Paul Steven Miller, The impact of assisted suicide on persons with disabilities—is it a right without freedom?, *Issues in Law & Medicine* 9:47, 54, 56 n. 33 (1993).

69. *See generally Report of Chairman Charles T. Canady to the Subcommittee on the Constitution of the Committee on the Judiciary of the House of Representatives* 104 Cong., 2d Sess., (September 1996).

70. *See, e.g.,* Brief for Amici Curiae, Gay Men's Health Crisis *et al.* in *Vacco v. Quill,* No. 95-1858, and *State of Washington v. Glucksberg,* No. 96-110, October Term, 1996, at p. 15.
71. For the Council's proposals as to how America might better afford people with disabilities opportunities for independence, dignity, self-sufficiency, and full participation, *see* National Council on Disability, *Achieving Independence: The Challenge for the 21st Century* (1996).